A HANDBOOK
FOR
IMPROVING YOUR DIET


Recipes, Charts and Tips
for a Smooth Transition
to Healthier Foods



by
Carol A. Nostrand

Printed in the United States of America
First Printing: May, 1985
Second Printing: June, 1985
Third Printing: February, 1986
Fourth Printing: February, 1988
Fifth Printing: January, 1990
Sixth Printing: February, 1992

ISBN: 0-9614721-0-3

Eatongude Press
259 West 4th Street, #19
New York, New York 10014

DEDICATION:

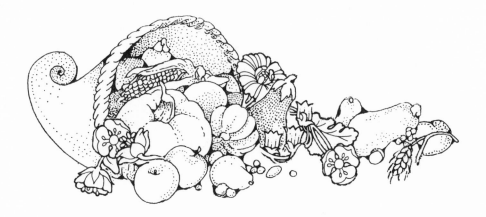

FOR ALL OF NATURE
SING WE OUR GRATEFUL PRAISE
TO THEE

ACKNOWLEDGEMENTS:

My special thanks to those who first encouraged me to write this book:

Charles C. Bell
Alan H. Nittler, M.D.
Leo Roy, M.D.

And to those who edited it and gave me their helpful critiques:

Sarah Bingham, M.A.
Michelle Harrison, M.D.
Barbara Friedlander Meyer
Marshall Nostrand
Neil S. Orenstein, Ph.D.
Richard Roberts
Jairo Rodriguez, D.C.
Sproutman

To Floyd D. Page, who graciously offered me the use of his word processor. Because of his generosity, patience and moral support, the three years of typing and editing was a joy.

To Eva Graf, who has taught me much about nutritional cooking, and who inspires me with the ease with which she creates delicious and nutritious goodies.

To my clients, who kept asking me when this book would be finished. It is their need that created it. I give it to them with love and gratitude.

---

******* TABLE OF CONTENTS *******

----------

SECTION II:
TIPS FOR MAKING A SMOOTH TRANSITION
TO HEALTHIER FOODS, pp.33-97.

----------

SECTION III:
RECIPES, pp.99-296.

----------------------------------------------

# TABLE OF CONTENTS, SECTION III, RECIPES

# TABLE OF CONTENTS, SECTION IV.

---

## SECTION IV:
## APPENDIX, FOOTNOTES, BIBLIOGRAPHY & INDEXES

------------------------------------------------

## INTRODUCTION

Why change your diet?

It may be because you are ill, and a dietary change has been recommended by your nutrition consultant or doctor.

Or, perhaps you have read that it can prevent illness later in life.

Or, perhaps you just don't feel as well as usual, and think that a better diet may help.

Or, you wish to lose or gain weight.

Or, a friend has changed his or her diet, and looks and feels much better.

Regardless of the reason, changing one's diet can present a confusing array of questions and conflicts.

We are used to eating certain foods. We know how to prepare them. We have our schedules and our life styles, and our diets fit into them. A change in diet often conjures up a threatening image of disruption and deprivation.

Your life does not need to be disrupted, and you do not need to be deprived of delicious goodies. With a few hints and guidelines and some easy, delicious recipes, a change in diet can be gradual, taking place with little stress. As the process unfolds, you will continuously be delighted with new taste treats which will more than replace your old favorites. As you make these discoveries, and find your own shortcuts, the process will become easier and more enjoyable.

Best of all, you will begin to experience increased health and vitality.

This book contains basic, practical information that can be helpful in making a transition to healthier foods, and delicious recipes that are highly nutritious and easy to prepare.

The book is divided into four sections.

The first section addresses the questions and conflicts most commonly faced when changing one's diet. The thought of these conflicts often prevents a change in diet, or can make a change more difficult. They are partially based on the <u>fear</u> of change, but they are real and important questions, and should be considered.

The second section of the book lists foods which support over all health, and those which do not, and contains practical methods for incorporating healthier foods into your life with ease.
This section also notes the types of foods necessary for a balanced diet, and how to combine them, and it contains lists, charts and other guidelines to help make a change with the least amount of stress.

The main portion, or third section, of the book contains recipes designed for great taste, simplicity in preparation, and maximum nutritional value. The foods used are vital foods - those which can aid any health maintenance or health regaining program. Many recipes are geared to one person, and can be easily multiplied. They are primarily milk and wheat free, since many people are allergic to wheat and milk.
In addition to the recipes, simple cooking techniques with lists of variations are included in each recipe section. This helps eliminate elaborate planning ahead and assists you in experimenting with your own recipes. This gives you more flexibility to shop and plan meals according to your taste, nutritional requirements, financial situation, the climate and availability of fresh foods, and all the other variables that change from day to day.

The recipes are not limited to one particular type of diet, since we are all at varying stages of transition. There are recipes familiar to more "conventional" cooking, including chicken and fish, and there are recipes for diets which emphasize raw food, or grains and beans. In brief, recipes to be enjoyed by anyone that prefers great taste, good nutrition, and simplicity in preparation.

The fourth section of the book contains an Appendix, Footnotes, a Bibliography, a Special Index and an Alphabetical Index.

The Appendix includes helpful reference material such as a "natural foods" glossary, natural foods kitchen hints, hints for cleaning utensils easily, a list of common food additives and their level of toxicity, and lists of "hidden" sugar and salt in processed foods.

The Appendix also includes a planned menu chart for one week, notes on planning menus, and approximately 50 meal suggestions. The list of meal suggestions is extensive in order to help you with your own meal planning, by illustrating the wide variety of possible combinations.

Footnoted references and a bibliography are also included for further exploration into nutritional data and delicious, healthful eating.

The Indexes list recipes alphabetically, and by category, such as "Snacks for Work or Travel", "Food for Children", "Allergy Free Recipes", and "Quick Foods". The Indexes are well detailed, not only to help you find information easily, but also to serve as reference guides in formulating your own recipes and meal plans from the vast quantity of information contained in this Handbook.

SECTION I

# OVERCOMING CONFLICTS IN CHANGING YOUR DIET

Changing one's diet is a an unfolding process of self-discovery, basically through trial and error, sometimes with the help of a nutrition consultant or doctor.

Profound and positive changes can take place mentally and emotionally, as well as physically, as your life style and mental clarity is affected by the new, vital foods. Change, even when positive, is still a shock to the system, and sometimes certain adjustments and compromises from time to time can help you adapt until you are able to make more drastic changes, which will come naturally.

A change of diet should be gradual. That is, do not try to go from a "meat and potato" to a totally raw food diet unless advised and guided by your nutrition consultant or doctor to do so. Your body -- physical, mental, emotional and spiritual -- needs a chance to make necessary adjustments at its own pace.

Each step will evolve naturally from the last. This gives your system and your life style time to adjust as you are ready. With a gradual transition you will also be less likely to become discouraged or bored with the new diet, and less likely to give it up, or to reject the changes it will make.

At the same time, exercise enough self discipline to avoid the foods which contribute to ill health. This is crucial to keep the process moving toward better health. The more assiduously you avoid these foods, the more quickly you will lose your taste for them, and the more quickly your body will maintain good health.

This section addresses the most common questions that arise when considering a change of diet. It helps to know that most of us are confronted with some of the same basic conflicts. Does this sound familiar?

"Would changing my diet really affect the quality of my health?

What would it mean to my life style? None of my friends eats that way. How could I go out to restaurants with them, or to their house for dinner? I don't want to be one of those fanatic "health nuts" who say they can't eat this or that.

Is it really worth all the changes I have to make?

Health foods are so expensive. How do you know that they're any better than the foods in my supermarket?

I don't have time to plan and prepare foods, either. I have a really busy schedule, especially in the morning.

What'll I do at work? There are no health food restaurants near me. Even if there were, they're too expensive to eat in every day. Could I take something with me to work? Like what?

I'm too tired at the end of the day to prepare a meal. I need to grab something quick. I don't know how to cook health foods. Besides, I hate to cook.

I know I should get a lot of variety in my diet, but I can't be bothered planning meals. It's so much easier eating the same foods over and over.

I only cook for myself, and it's so boring to prepare a meal for one person.

(or)

I cook for my family. They'll never eat this way, and I don't want to prepare different meals for everybody.

I'm already depressed from not feeling well. Now, on top of that, do I have to give up all my favorite foods? Are there really foods that are good for me that taste as good as my favorites?"

These are all good questions. The answers aren't the same for everyone. Each of you will find your own solutions as you go through the process, but perhaps some of the discoveries my clients and I have made can be helpful.

One important common denominator for anyone changing their diet: a sense of humor. Don't be obsessive with the change. Find your own balance between being "light" with yourself, and pushing against your resistance to positive change. Keep the momentum going through self-discipline, self-respect, and self-love.

CHAPTER 1

THE "STRANGE" NEW WORLD OF HEALTH FOODS

Eating "health food" does not mean taking away all the good things, and eating foods that are "strange" and boring, but good for you.

It means eating many of the same foods you love, but in a whole state - fresh fruits and vegetables, whole grains, beans, nuts and seeds, certain meat and dairy products and certain sweets. It may also mean simply changing your emphasis - eating less meat, dairy and sweets, and more fresh fruits and vegetables, whole grains, beans and nuts and seeds.

It means discovering the marvelous variety of delicious fruits and vegetables, including more of them in your diet, and preparing them with as little heat as possible, so that they retain their bright color, deep flavor, fiber, and nutrients.

It means enjoying your pasta and bread, while getting a health return from them, by eating them in a whole grain state instead of a refined, or processed state. With whole grains, the outer layer (or "bran") and the inner core (or "germ") of the grain has not been processed out, so you get fiber, B vitamins, vitamin E, protein and minerals along with a delicious nutty flavor that is absent in the processed grain.

The world of health foods may seem strange or new because some of these unprocessed foods are unfamiliar to you, but they certainly were not strange to our ancestors. They are foods which have supported life for generations.

Another reason eating health foods often seems "strange" is because it may mean changing some old habits. You may need to change the proportion of foods you eat - perhaps less red meat, less sweets, and more vegetables. You may need to find new stores, new ways of preparing foods, and different brands that are less processed and free of salt and sugar. The thought of the initial effort in changing old routines can lock you into bad habits, eating foods which ultimately can cause more stress. We have enough stress in our lives without eating foods which contribute to stress. At least this is one area over which we have some control, and it can be the most enjoyable!

Once you have incorporated healthier foods into your daily routine and found your own short cuts, shopping and preparation will be easy. You'll find that it takes no more time to lightly steam fresh vegetables than to warm up frozen or canned vegetables, to make whole grain pasta or bread instead of refined. Even brown rice takes only 1/2 hour, and the nutritional value in these unprocessed foods will give you additional health support.

A small portion of foods within the range of "health foods" has come to us from other cultures. These foods can add health benefits and delicious taste variation to our recipes, but we might avoid using them because they are different. They are not foods we were brought up on, so the taste, texture, preparation and association is not familiar to us. This is one of the strongest reasons we resist changing our diets and the introduction of new foods. This is a very natural reaction. Many emotions are connected to our food, but try not to allow that to limit you in choosing foods you may love.

It is helpful to know something about the food, and then to introduce it gradually by including it in familiar types of recipes.

Following are some of the foods included in "health food" cooking, and in this book, which may be unfamiliar to you. Refer to the "Glossary" for more detailed information on each of these foods.

Agar Agar: A jelling agent, like gelatin.

Arrowroot: A thickener used like cornstarch.

Carob: A bean, ground into a powder and used in place of chocolate.

Miso: Soy bean paste, used to add a deep, salty flavor to soups, sauces, etc.

Tahini: Sesame seed butter. It's something like peanut butter, but it's made with sesame seeds instead of peanuts.

Tamari: Soy sauce, used to add a deep, salty flavor and dark color to sauces, etc.

Tofu: Soy bean curd. Used in numerous ways as a protein, and in place of dairy.

Your recipes can be greatly enhanced by using different kinds of foods. Keep expanding, introducing new foods and new types of recipes. Allow yourself time to get to know the food, and to enjoy your discoveries.

CHAPTER 2

COST & SPOILAGE

In some cases, health foods cost more, simply because they spoil faster without the addition of toxic preservatives.

When you consider the cost of good food, take into account the quality of the foods, and the quality of health they reflect in your body. Good foods are an investment in your future -- preventive "medicine".

Junk filler foods are also expensive, however, especially since they are consumed fast. The sugar, salt and additives in them stimulate cravings for more, so you buy more. Eating more nutritious foods tends to satisfy faster than empty foods, so that one tends to be less likely to crave more. Healthy snacks, such as fresh or dried fruit, or nuts and seeds, though expensive, satisfy in smaller amounts, and limit over-eating by their very expense.

If you have the space, certain foods, such as whole grains and beans can be purchased in bulk to cut down on cost.

Naturally, with fresh foods and those with no preservatives there is greater chance for spoilage. This is especially a concern for small households. Fresh fruits and vegetables will need to be purchased more often, but sometimes they can be bought in smaller packages. If not, extra amounts need not go to waste. For example, leafy greens, such as lettuce or parsley, can be made into a delicious "green drink", and vegetables can be juiced. See Recipe section.

In addition, there are many tips to help avoid spoilage. See "Natural Food Kitchen Hints" and "Shopping Hints".

Keep in mind that GOOD FOOD TASTES BETTER!

CHAPTER 3


AVAILABILITY OF FOODS


Most "health foods" are easily available, since fresh fruits and vegetables, some whole grains and beans and nuts and seeds can be purchased at your local market.

In discussing quality health foods and their availability, it is necessary to use a good-better-best guide. The highest quality health foods are the least processed - those closest to their natural state. In this case, the best source is your own farm, where you can pick organically grown fruits and vegetables fresh. Next best is a local organic farm, then a good health food store, food co-op or fruit and vegetable market.

If you are limited to shopping in a supermarket, read labels, become thoroughly aware of what you are buying, and demand the best quality from your supermarket. Find out when fruits and vegetables are delivered to the store and how long they have been on the truck, so that you can purchase them as fresh as possible. (Refer to "Kitchen Hints" for tips on keeping foods fresh.)

Familiarize yourself with the most common toxic food additives, and with products that contain "hidden" sugar and salt. Refer to the "Appendix" for lists of these additives and products. Take copies of these lists with you to the store.

If you cannot get the purest of foods, don't worry over them! Clean them as best you can (See "Kitchen Hints", pp.299-301.), then relax and enjoy them.

Following is a chart showing where you can purchase "health food".

AVAILABILITY CHART

| PRODUCT | SHOPPING SOURCE | | |
|---|---|---|---|
| | SUPER MARKET | HEALTH FOOD STORE | SPECIALTY MARKET |
| Fresh Fruit & Vegetables | * | * | * |
| Sprouts | * | * | * |
| Sea Vegetables | | * | * |
| Whole Wheat Bread | * | * | * |
| 100% Rye Bread | | * | * |
| Essene Bread | | * | |
| Whole Wheat Noodles | * | * | * |
| Buckwheat Noodles | | * | * |
| Brown Rice | * | * | * |
| Barley | * | * | * |
| Bulgar | * | * | * |
| Buckwheat (Kasha) | * | * | * |
| Millet | | * | * |
| Wheat or Rye Berries | | * | * |
| Whole Wheat or Rye Flour | * | * | * |
| Rice,Soy or Millet Flour | | * | * |
| Cornmeal | * | * | * |
| Lentils or Split Peas | * | * | * |
| Aduki Beans | | * | * |
| Black,Kidney, etc.Beans | * | * | * |
| Sugar-Free Granola | * | * | * |
| Rolled Oats | * | * | * |
| Popcorn | * | * | * |
| Eggs | * | * | * |
| Organic Eggs | | * | * |
| Meat | * | * | * |
| Organic Meat | | * | * |
| Nuts and Seeds | * | * | * |
| Unsulfured Dried Fruit | | * | * |
| Tahini, Miso, Tofu | | * | * |
| Kuzu, Agar Agar | | * | * |
| Soy Sauce, Barley Malt | | * | * |
| Raw Honey, Carob Powder | | * | * |
| Pure Maple Syrup,Molasses | * | * | * |
| Apple Cider Vinegar | * | * | * |
| Olive Oil | * | * | * |
| Cold Pressed Oils | | * | * |
| Sugar-Free Condiments | | * | |
| Sugar-Free Juice | | * | |
| Distilled or Spring Water | * | * | |
| Herb Tea | * | * | * |
| Grain Coffee Substitutes | *(Postum) | * | * |
| Yogurt | * | * | * |
| Cayenne Pepper | * | * | * |
| Vegetable Salt Substitutes | | * | |

Note: Specialty market includes oriental markets, fruit and vegetable markets, farms, meat or fish markets, etc.

CHAPTER 4

GETTING TO KNOW THE HEALTH FOOD STORE

Since the main portion of "health foods" consists of fresh fruits and vegetables, and whole grains and beans, they do not necessarily have to be purchased in a health food store. However, the health food store does contain good quality whole grains and beans, nuts and seeds, organic eggs and sometimes organic meats, fruits and vegetables, as well as unprocessed, chemical and sugar free oils and condiments. (Organic meat and eggs are from animals raised free-range, fed on their natural feed rather than chemicals, without being injected with hormones and antibiotics.) In addition, health food stores contain a wide variety of delicious, "new" foods such as tahini or miso.

Health food stores may feel intimidating at first - a maze of unfamiliar foods, and a new language of nutrition, often associated with "health nuts" and faddism. We get used to the routine of going to certain stores. We are familiar with the aisles, the smells, the clerks and people that shop there, as well as the types of food.

Approach your health food store with an open mind. Try not to attach any negative associations to it, and don't be afraid of it. Consult friends, a nutritionist, and store clerks for the best brands to buy. Take along the "List of Staples" as a guide.

At first, just explore the health food store for the fun of it. Read labels, because not everything in a health food store is healthy. Pick up a couple of items you would normally use - perhaps a delicious jam made with honey and no preservatives, a pure ice cream, a loaf of whole grain bread, or a box of whole grain, sugar-free cereal.

After you feel more comfortable, you may find yourself looking around more, noticing new foods. Read their labels. Ask about them and how they are used. It is a process of developing new relationships in your life. It will happen naturally, if you allow it. Eventually your health food store will be an old friend.

CHAPTER 5

PREPARATION TIME

Very few of us have time to spend hours planning and preparing a meal. In fact, many people find that they expend so much energy in their jobs and other daily activities that even the thought of planning a meal, looking up recipes, and shopping for specific ingredients causes stress, especially when the recipes and ingredients are unfamiliar.

There are several ways you can cut down on "preparation stress":

A. Set up your kitchen so that the preparation flows more easily. Make sure you have good counter space, with a cutting board, and easy access to pots, utensils and spices that you use frequently. Give yourself the gift of basic equipment and utensils that will make your life easier. (See "Utensils and Equipment", pp.68-71.)

B. Keep on hand some basic food staples that store well, and which can be used in a variety of ways to create whole meals. (See the list of staples, pp.74-76, and "Natural Food Kitchen Hints", pp.299-301 for tips on storage.)

C. Get to know the basic food types you need in a day to provide you with a balanced diet. This gives you an over-all format within which to work.

D. Learn a few basic, simple cooking techniques that are especially quick and easy, but which allow for variety, expansion and creativity. In this way you can be as simple or as elaborate as you have the time, energy or inspiration to be.

Knowledge of a few techniques eliminates the need for excessive planning ahead, for using recipes, or for shopping for specific ingredients. Instead, having a technical framework within which to work frees you to create recipes that fit your mood and/or nutritional needs, and to use foods which are fresh, already on hand, or easy to find.

Specific techniques, rather than specific recipes, also provide greater opportunity for variety, which is so important for a balanced diet.

Some examples of foods prepared with simple cooking techniques are blended soups, "basic soups", blended cereals, nut milks, grain pilaf, quick blended sauces, quick steam soup or meal, meal-in-one sauté and easy salad. For a description of these techniques, see p.96. The Recipe Section also includes a description of each technique, with lists of suggested ingredients, plus a few examples.

E. Become familiar with recipes that require very little time to plan or prepare, such as those in this book. Refer to the Index for a list of recipes which are especially quick (See pp.338-339.).

F. Although it is always best to prepare foods fresh (which is one of the advantages in using quick, basic cooking techniques), some foods store fairly well pre-prepared and kept in the refrigerator or freezer. Again, work with the "good, better, best guide". It's better to eat something prepared the night before than to grab "junk" food.

In deciding which foods to prepare ahead and store, choose those that store well, and are versatile in their uses. This helps avoid boredom with eating the same food two or three days in a row. (Try not to eat foods beyond three days in a row, however. Variety is important for a balanced diet, and it is possible to manifest an allergic reaction to a food eaten too much, too often. See "Allergens", p.55.)

Examples of foods which can be prepared ahead are as follows:

(1) Spreads, dressings or dips, such as miso-tahini spread (p.209), tofu dip (p. 205), or tahini dip (p.206). These keep well for several days stored in covered glass jars in the refrigerator. Add water to them and they become sauces or dressings. See each recipe for their many uses.

(2) Sunburgers (p.230) and Lentil Walnut Burgers (p.273) keep well in the freezer. They're good hot or cold as a snack, a meal, or to take to work.

(3) Brown rice or other grains. Cooked brown rice stores quite well, and can be used in a variety of ways. (See Recipe Section for details.) Blend it with hot water as a cereal; add it to soups; lightly sauté it by itself or with other foods; put it into loaves, etc.

(4) Cooked beans can be kept in the freezer or refrigerator. They can be added to vegetable soups or salads, made into burgers, or blended with hot water for a creamy bean soup, sauce or dip;

(5) Cooked chicken can be diced and added to cold salads, soups, vegetable dishes, made into curried chicken, etc.

(6) Sauerkraut can be eaten as is, added to salads, baked with potatoes, etc.

(7) Leafy greens, such as lettuce, parsley, watercress, or swiss chard, can be washed, cut up and kept in a plastic lettuce container. They are then ready to add to salads, vegetable loaves or green drinks.*

(8) Raw vegetables can be washed, chopped and refrigerated, ready to add to salads, soups, vegetable dishes, juices, or as snacks with dips.*

* Please note that washing or slicing vegetables and greens ahead of time results in extreme loss of nutrients, so in general it is not advised. Again, use the "good-better-best" guide.


As you become familiar with the cooking techniques, with "new" foods, and with the recipes in this book, food preparation will become easier and take less time. You will begin to find ways of making your own adjustments and shortcuts. It is a process of learning and discovery. Take your time, incorporating new techniques as you are ready. Enjoy it well!

CHAPTER 6

RESTAURANT EATING

Usually, we associate eating out with relaxing, enjoying ourselves, and eating what most appeals to us on the menu. The foods with appeal are sometimes those that do not support over-all health and vitality - those that are "creamy, gooey, fatty or fried." We need to change our associations, and break our habits of choosing foods which put stress on our bodies, and which ultimately limit our enjoyment. We usually choose the same restaurants, and the same foods on the menu. Begin to look at menus with a "different" eye, and you will see that there really are foods you can eat.

Appetizers are usually foods you can enjoy, such as freshly made soups, poached salmon, artichokes, salads, or steamed vegetables. Some people enjoy a meal of just appetizers.

For an entrée, most restaurants offer fresh fish, lamb, baked chicken or other fowl as well as lightly steamed vegetables, baked potatoes and salads, and sometimes whole grains.

When choosing from entrées, avoid dishes that are high in fat, or are overly cooked, fried (such as tempura or fried chicken), heavily salted or sugared, or drenched in rich sauces or thick, gooey cheese. In some restaurants, it is possible to ask that the sauce be put on the side, or that the food be cooked without fat. Many restaurants are now accustomed to such requests, and are able to fulfill them.

It may also be wise to avoid pork or shellfish, which are often contaminated.

Usually the dessert is the worst offender in restaurants. Order fresh fruit, or have your dessert at home. Or, "restaurant hop". Have your dessert at a health food restaurant, where you can order a dessert made without processed flour or sugar. Restaurant hopping also gives you time to digest your main course before having your dessert.

If you eat at "better" restaurants, you are more likely to get fresh, good quality food, freshly made and not over-cooked. (This is not necessarily a "health food" restaurant, which often emphasizes cheese and wheat in their dishes.) To cut down on the cost of a better restaurant, avoid the "x-tras", which put additional stress on the body, and which limit the digestion of your meal - excessive alcohol, sugary desserts, coffee, teas containing caffeine or tannin.

Don't stuff yourself. Light eating is easier on the digestion as well as the pocket book. If the portions are more than you can eat, take the rest home! You'll get two or three meals for the price of one.

Sometimes it helps to eat a small portion of something at home, before you go to a reataurant. This may sound silly, but it serves several purposes:

1. When you are less hungry, your will power is stronger. You are less likely to order large amounts of food. Large amounts are usually poor combinations of food, as well as too much to eat for ease of digestion.

2. By ordering less, you'll spend less, yet still have the pleasure of dining out with friends.

3. By spending less, you can choose a finer restaurant with better quality food and more pleasant atmosphere.

4. If you are with friends who do not eat as you do, and you go to a restaurant you would not normally pick, which has a limited menu, you won't mind eating less as much as you would if you were extra hungry. Usually a delicious appetizer and one or two special side dishes are plenty to eat and nutritionally perfect.

5. If the menu is limited, and you need to order less, and your friends wonder why, you won't have to explain much. Both of you will be more at ease if you truthfully can say that what you have ordered is perfect.

6. When you are less famished, and your will power is greater, you are more likely to order foods which are right for you to eat rather than the less nutritious foods with an "emotional pull".

Some suggestions of foods you can eat before you go out are baked squash, baked potato, raw vegetables with a dip, artichoke, soup, yogurt or fruit.

Eating out is usually a festive occasion, a time for being with friends. Eating well can only add to your enjoyment.

CHAPTER 7

FOODS TO GO FOR WORK OR TRAVEL

When traveling or going to work, take along any of the following:
    Nuts and seeds
    Soaked dried fruit
    Fresh fruit and vegetables
    Pure juices
    Soups in a thermos, or soup bouillon
        cubes or powders to be mixed with
        hot water
    Herb tea bags
    Whole grain breads and crackers
    Home made granola or granola bought in
        a health food store

    See the "Special Index", "Snacks to Go for Work or Travel", p.337, for a complete list of ideas.
    Snacks can be carried in baggies and/or small plastic containers, wide-mouthed thermos bottles, mason jars, etc. Canvas carrying bags with a shoulder strap, lined with washable, water-resistant fabric or plastic, can be purchased or made.
    Sometimes left-overs can be used, or "Quick Foods" can be prepared in the morning.
    When traveling, stopping at a roadside restaurant is often a welcome break, and yet the menu is often less than desirable. If you have munched on good snacks along the way, at least you won't be so hungry that you'll feel the need to order something you may regret later. Most roadside restaurants have soups, and many have salad bars which range from adequate to excellent.

CHAPTER 8

COOKING FOR OTHERS

Cooking for family and friends can present a whole new set of challenges.

At the same time, it gives you the opportunity to introduce your family to more delicious recipes, and gives you the pleasure of feeding them foods which support their good health.

Usually, if you just prepare what you love, it will be a huge success with everyone. (Warning: Don't tell them you are feeding them "health food". Just tell them it's a new recipe you are trying.)

In some cases, it may be better at first to use familiar recipes they enjoy, but with "health-full" changes. Following are a few ideas which will be discussed and illustrated more fully in Section II.

A. Convert recipes, substituting "health-full" ingredients for stressful ones. For example, use whole grain flour in place of white flour. Use honey in place of sugar. Use brown rice in place of white rice. (See "Conversion", pp.62-66.)

Sometimes the conversion can take place gradually. For example, at first use a combination of whole grain flour with white flour or brown rice with white rice, or whole grain noodles with processed noodles. Increase the proportion of whole grain to processed as you and your family are ready.

B. Supplement recipes, adding nutritious ingredients to your present recipes. (See "Supplements", p.67.)

C. Use recipes that are the same types of foods as those your family enjoys. For example, make sunburgers instead of hamburgers, and use a sugar and chemical free ketchup on top. Make cookies and candies out of whole grains, nuts and seeds, honey and dried fruit instead of white flour and sugar.

Other good recipes for family and guests who are accustomed to "traditional" American cuisine are the following: (See "Recipes").

Appetizers: mixed raw vegetables with "Spring Green Dip"; "Vegetable Soup"; "Potato Leek Soup", artichokes.

Main Course: "Coq au Vin"; any of the fish recipes; "Broccoli Quiche".

Dessert: "Zucchini Bread"; "Fresh Fruit Ice Cream", strawberries with carob sauce.

D. Explore the health food store and purchase products which resemble those your family enjoys. For example, there are delicious whole grain cereals, breads and condiments such as jellies, mayonnaise and ketchup that are made without sugar or toxic additives. There is ice cream and soft drinks made without sugar, - even beer made without alcohol.

E. When cooking for children, have them share in the preparation. Children usually enjoy helping prepare meals when it is treated as something fun you are doing together, rather than a chore. And, they appreciate the food more.

Teach them how to grow sprouts. Children love to grow sprouts, and usually love to eat them. Include sprouts as much as possible in their meals, particularly since they usually don't enjoy salads.

Children are more likely to eat raw vegetables if given to them in small pieces to munch on. Perhaps give them a dip they enjoy, too. Blend cottage cheese in a blender, or use any of the recipes in this book. Or, use almond butter purchased in a health food store, or made at home.

Another way to give children vegetables is in the form of juices - freshly juiced.

At party time, or whenever you feel inspired, you can arrange chopped vegetables or fruits in designs and funny faces. For example, cherry tomatoes for eyes, 1/2 sliced green pepper for ears, sliced mushrooms for a nose, a slice of beet for a mouth with corn for teeth, and celery leaves or parsley for hair.

There are many desserts and snacks that your children will love, which will nourish them at the same time, such as fresh fruit ice cream, nut/seed candies, etc. See the Recipe Section and the "Special Index", p.340 for a complete list of "Foods Children Love."


Make any changes gradually. Don't worry, your family and friends will love the new recipes. They are delicious, and your guests will feel better eating them.

CHAPTER 9


## VISITING FAMILY AND FRIENDS


From time to time you may be the brunt of some teasing. This is especially difficult with family, since loved ones may feel that your new diet is a rejection of them, and an attack on your upbringing. You have to decide how much you can share about your new understandings and how much you can compromise in eating with them. Tension created in certain situations can create more stress in your body than any foods.

If you decide it is best to share their meal, relax and enjoy it, fully digest the love that went into preparing it for you, and enjoy the company!

There are times when you can offer to prepare a meal for others. This is a good opportunity to introduce them to your new way of eating, but use recipes that are not too different from theirs. (For a few examples, see "Cooking for Others", p.25.) Remember that your way is not necessarily right for them.

You could also bring something with you for dessert, or snack. A few examples of house gifts are Sunny Snack, p.278; Oatmeal Cookies, p.283; a pure honey vanilla ice cream with a jar of carob mint sauce, p.296; zucchini bread, p.125, or gingered carrot marmalade, p.212. You could package the gifts with ribbons, attractive labels, dried or fresh flowers, etc.

If you decide not to eat with family or friends, try not to explain too much, as it usually complicates matters. You can always say that you have discovered that certain foods do not agree with you, or that your doctor or nutritionist has you on a restricted diet. Usually, the less you say, the better.

The most difficult times will be when you yourself doubt the validity of your new regime. Most people go through periods when, as their bodies release toxins, they experience discomfort. If you are not sure what this discomfort is, check with your nutrition consultant or doctor, and don't give up. The crisis will pass and you will be stronger in mind and body than before.

Eventually your family and friends will get used to your new way of eating. Just love them, and let them know you are not judging their diet. They will eventually accept the new healthier you.

CHAPTER 10

FOOD CRAVINGS

Food cravings can indicate many things.
They can be because your body lacks nutrients. If you eat nutrient-poor foods, your body will continuously send out signals for more food until it is satisfied. Eating nutrient-rich foods, therefore, can help prevent cravings.

Cravings for sweet or salty foods can be an indication of a blood sugar imbalance, which can result from excesses of sugar or nutrient poor foods, stress, emotional trauma, inherent weakness, etc. In this case, it would probably be best to avoid all sweets, including honey, molasses, maple syrup, and dried fruit, until the blood sugar imbalance is corrected. Otherwise, even these natural sweets can trigger a sugar binge similar to an alcoholic's craving for alcohol. This situation, which is quite common, should be under the care of a nutrition consultant or doctor.

Cravings for sweet foods can also be stimulated by consuming an excess of salty foods, and vice versa. This is the body's attempt to balance these excesses. Moderation in eating such foods is important.

Cravings can be clues to food sensitivities. Sometimes we crave the very foods to which we are allergic. This can apply even to the foods from the "Foods to Enjoy" list. (See pp.36-46. Also see "Allergens", "Foods to Avoid", p.55.) Eating the allergen stops the craving and gives you an initial high. Unfortunately, it results in a let-down later and contributes to further breakdown of the body. It is similiar to an alcoholic addiction. The craving is stimulated by withdrawal symptoms which are postponed by eating the food.'

Food cravings can be the result of dehydration. Sometimes we eat foods when we are actually thirsty. Very often, people who are overweight find that drinking more water (and eating nutrient-rich foods) helps reduce their desire for food.

Food cravings can also be from lack of oxygen in the body, and from blocked, frustrated creative energy. Deep breathing, and finding positive outlets for your creativity can help.

There is a great deal of emotional attachment to food, as well. This is a subject for an entire book itself, beyond the scope of this book. To touch on it briefly, however, there is, for example, often a connection between sugar and reward, love or approval. Food becomes a substitute for love and nourishment on a deep level. The pain of the emotions connected with the lack of love, including self-love and a spiritual awareness, is suppressed by eating the food. Examine your attachments to food closely. If you can avoid the food, and allow yourself to become in touch with, and experience the emotions, you can learn a great deal about yourself, and help yourself release the need for the food.

You will find that as you eliminate one undesirable food from your diet, you will lose your appreciation for another that you thought would be difficult to give up. As the body cleanses itself of toxic matter, it becomes more sensitive to the taste and effect of food. Devitalized food will taste dead, sugar will seem too sweet, coffee will have too strong an effect, etc.

Remember the "good, better, best" guide. Find a "good" substitute for the food you crave and eat that for a while. Then substititute that for a "better" food, and eventually eat the "best" foods. Use the "Transition Chart" (p.59) and "Conversion" rules (pp.62-66) to help you choose your substitutes.

For example, substitute a carob bar (without sugar) for chocolate. After a short time, switch to home-made carob candies, since many of the store bought carob bars contain oils which are difficult to digest. Then, eat fruit instead of candies.

Another example: substitute water-processed decaffeinated coffee for regular coffee. (Other decaffeinated coffees contain high levels of metals used in the processing.) After a short time switch to pure grain beverages, such as Pero or Cafix, and to herb teas.

Another example: Have sugar-free ice cream in place of ice cream with sugar or chemicals. Then switch to ice creams made from fresh fruit without dairy (p.294).

If you have a craving for a food that seems healthy to you, try it and note your reaction. If it is from the list of "Foods to Enjoy", it could be something you lack and you will feel better eating it - not just right away, but for hours afterward.

Discuss your cravings with your nutrition consultant or physician. Eventually you will be able to distinguish between what is a craving for an allergen and what you are actually lacking.

If you give in to a craving and eat something you are trying to give up, examine how you felt before and after. Record any negative reactions you had (but don't expect them), then resolve to be stronger next time. Each time it will be easier to exercise more self control. As your body becomes less toxic, the cravings will become less and less and finally will fall away.

SECTION II:

## MAKING A SMOOTH TRANSITION TO HEALTHIER FOODS

Our bodies are constantly striving for health. Any health regaining program has the same basic principle - that of:
(1) rebuilding the weak organs and tissues and replenishing the body with all needed essential proteins, vitamins, minerals, oils and enzymes; and,
(2) detoxifying the body, or getting rid of toxic waste that has caused an imbalance, or has prevented the body from functioning to its fullest capacity.

Food is a vital and very basic part of any health regaining program since, ideally, it helps regenerate our body structures through its nourishing properties, and aids in the elimination of toxic matter.
There are certain foods which generally support the life-giving process, and there are certain foods which inhibit this process, causing further stress and contributing to physical and mental breakdown.

In general, the foods you choose should be as close to their natural state as possible. They should be whole, unprocessed, and without toxic additives. The closer foods are to the state in which they grew, the more vitality they contain and will transfer to you.

Meal planning, preparation and consumption of foods should be geared toward maximum preservation and assimilation of nutrients as well as great taste.

Each of us has special needs, both nutritional and practical, which affect the foods we choose and the ways in which we plan and prepare our meals. For everyone, good taste, simplicity in preparation and a diet that is healthy and fits into one's life style is essential.

A change of diet must, therefore, be as smooth, as delicious and as easily workable as possible while still maintaining good nutrition.

This section will present guidelines which can be helpful in making a smooth transition to a better diet geared to individual needs. The following points will be considered:

FOODS WHICH GENERALLY SUPPORT GOOD HEALTH, AND THOSE WHICH ENCOURAGE ILL HEALTH (CHAPTERS 1 AND 2).

HOW TO GO ABOUT MAKING A CHANGE WITH LITTLE STRESS (CHAPTERS 3-4).

HOW TO MAKE A DIET PRACTICAL AND EASILY WORKABLE, WITHOUT SACRIFICING GOOD TASTE AND NUTRITION (CHAPTERS 5-10).

CHAPTER 1

CHOOSING FOODS FOR HEALTH

The foods which most support over-all health are whole grains, nuts and seeds, sprouts, beans and peas, fresh fruits and vegetables, eggs, certain meat, fish and dairy products, certain oils, sweeteners and seasonings, fresh fruit and vegetable juices, herb teas, and pure water.

All of these foods will be most delicious and nutritious if they are as unadulterated, as fresh and as whole as possible.

******** FOODS TO ENJOY ********

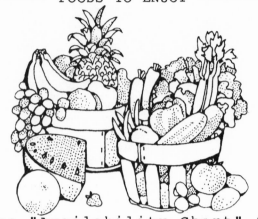

Note: See "Availability Chart" (p.14) for Sources for these "Foods to Enjoy".

WHOLE GRAINS
AND NOODLES, FLOUR & GRAIN SPROUTS

| | | |
|---|---|---|
| whole wheat | brown rice | barley |
| cornmeal | millet | rye |
| bulghur (cracked wheat) | | oats |
| buckwheat and kasha (buckwheat groats) | | |

Whole grains have protein, unsaturated fat, carbohydrates, vitamins, such as vitamins B and E, and minerals, such as phosphorus, iron and potassium.[1] They also contain fiber, an important aid to healthy elimination.[2]

The high nutrient value and fiber in whole grains help balance the metabolism, so they are less likely to contribute to weight imbalance than processed grains.[3]

Vary your grains as much as possible to get more nutrients and avoid "allergic" reactions (see "Foods to Avoid - Allergens").

Combining grains with beans or nuts and seeds increases their net protein utilized. (See Protein Combining).[4]

Refrigerate grains to keep them fresh. Whenever possible, grind your flour fresh.

To preserve nutrients and vitality in grains, prepare them with low heat. (See "Grains" in Recipe section.)[5]

Whole grains have a delicious, nutty flavor that is absent in processed grains.

## SPROUTS
(SPROUTED NUTS, SEEDS, BEANS OR GRAINS)

| alfalfa | buckwheat | lentil |
| sunflower | mung | chia |
| pumpkin | wheat | oat |
| rye | fenugreek | |

Since sprouts are still growing, they contain more vitality than any other food. They are good sources of protein, many vitamins and minerals, and fiber.[1]

See "Sprouts" in the Recipe Section.

## BEANS AND PEAS (LEGUMES)
AND THEIR FLOUR AND SPROUTS

| aduki | kidney | mung |
| garbanzo | lentil | soy |
| split peas | pinto | black |
| great white northern | | |

Beans and peas are good sources of protein, vitamins, such as B vitamins, and minerals, such as iron.[1]

Sprouting them increases their nutrient value and makes them easier to digest.[2]

Combining beans and peas with grains or nuts and seeds increases their net protein utilization (See Protein Combining.).[3]

## NUTS & SEEDS
## AND NUT BUTTERS & NUT MILKS (See "Beverages")

| | | |
|---|---|---|
| flax seeds | sesame seeds | almonds |
| pumpkin seeds | sunflower seeds | walnuts |
| pecans | brazil nuts | filberts |

chia seeds (seeds of the sage brush - high
    in protein)

Other nuts are good, but these are the best. Peanuts, which are not a nut but a legume, are, as with most legumes, difficult for many people to digest. In addition, they are a common allergen,[1] and often contain a mold, which has been found to be carcino-genic.[2] For a delicious nut butter, use almond or sesame seed butter (tahini).

Nuts and seeds, and "butters" and "milks" made from nuts and seeds, are high in calories, or "food energy", are rich sources of vitamins, such as B and E, of minerals, such as calcium, iron, potassium and magnesium, and of protein, and quality oil.[3]

Nuts and seeds, as with all oil-rich foods become rancid easily in processing, such as grinding, or by exposure to warm temperatures. Since rancid oils are extremely toxic, be sure to refrigerate all nuts and seeds. If you grind them, use them immediately, or keep them in the freezer for a short period of time. Off-taste can indicate rancidity. Fresh nuts and seeds have a sweeter taste and leave no bitter after-taste.

## EGGS

Eggs are a good source of complete protein, and contain vitamins, such as A, B, D and E, and minerals, such as selenium, zinc, sulfur and lecithin.[1]

Protein and other nutrients in eggs are more fully assimilated when eggs are eaten raw or lightly cooked (soft boiled or poached).[2] However, moderate your intake of raw eggs. When eaten in great quantity, they can inhibit the assimilation of biotin, one of the B vitamins.[3]

Use organic eggs, if possible. These are eggs from organically raised chicken. Non-organic eggs usually contain chemical residue such as hormones and antibiotics from the non-organically raised hens.[4]

Most researchers feel that eggs are not a major cause of cholesterol build up. In fact, eggs contain lecithin, which helps liquify cholesterol.[5] Many scientists feel that a primary cause of cholesterol build up is the lack of fiber and lack of essential nutrients in a diet of processed foods.[6]

The amount of eggs in the diet depends on the individual. Consult with your nutrition consultant or doctor.


FISH

Deep ocean fish          Pure-lake fish

Fish are a good source of protein, quality oil, vitamins and minerals, especially iodine and potassium.[1]

Limit shell fish such as lobster, clams, scallops, shrimp and oysters. They are difficult to digest and often contaminated.[2]

See "Fish" under "Recipes" for types of fish that are especially good to use.

## MEAT

Chicken                    Lamb

Meat is a source of protein, certain vitamins, such as B vitamins, and minerals, such as iron and phosphorus.[1]

When possible, use organically raised chicken. They are free of hormones, antibiotics and other chemicals. (See p.52.) Organic meat is more tender, less fatty and much more delicious.[2] When organic meats are not available, kosher meat is next best for being tender and tasty.

Lamb, although high in fat, is less full of hormones and antibiotics than other red meats. For those who prefer not to eliminate red meat for a while, lamb can be a "transition" meat.


## DAIRY

Certified raw, if possible:
   Goat milk
   unsalted butter
   yogurt
   kefir drink (like "liquified yogurt")
   cheeses that break easily: cottage, feta,
      pot, goat, kefir cheese (which is like
      sour cream), farmers cheese

Cow's milk is more commonly allergenic than goat's milk, and therefore should be limited if not eliminated. Pasteurization and homogenization make it still more difficult to digest, encouraging allergic reactions and mucous buildup.[1] Certified raw cow's milk is a first step in "transition" away from milk.

Use butter in moderation. Use unsalted butter that has no added dye. Butter yellow dye has been found to be cancer causing.[2]

## OILS

olive oil
"cold pressed" sesame, sunflower, flax
seed, soy, almond, avocado and walnut.
unsalted butter (raw, if possible)

"Cold pressed" oils are those which have
been extracted from the nut, seed or bean
with low heat and with no chemicals,
bleaching or deodorizing. They can be
purchased in health food stores. The label
will read "cold pressed".

Oils should be refrigerated to avoid
rancidity. If you rarely use them, store them
in the freezer, refrigerating a small amount.

Adding 200-400 I.U. of Vitamin E oil to
your oils can help protect them against
oxidation which leads to rancidity.[1]

When cooking with oils, use very low
heat and use olive oil or butter, since they
will not break down and become toxic on high
heats as easily as other oils.

For some people, soy oil on an ongoing
basis can be congesting, since it is a common
allergen.[2] Vary it with other oils.

Vary your oils as much as possible to
get a fuller range of essential fatty acids
and nutrients.

## BEVERAGES

water
nut milk or grain water
pure fruit or vegetable juice
certified raw cow's milk or goat milk

Drink 6-8 glasses of water a day. Preferably use spring water, or (if recommended
by your nutrition consultant or doctor),
distilled water.

## VEGETABLES

Vegetables are good sources of vitamins, such as A, C and B; of minerals, such as potassium, magnesium, iron and calcium; of amino acids and water. Raw vegetables are one of our best sources of fiber.

The leafy greens are especially high in vitamins C, A and B, in iron and calcium, and in chlorophyll, which is an important blood-builder. Include them in your diet daily.[1]

Sea vegetables, or sea weeds, are extremely rich in minerals, especially iodine.[2] They can be purchased dried in a whole or powdered form. You may need to become accustomed to their sea-weed flavor and association, but once you have, they can be an important adjunct to a nutritionally sound and tasty diet. Try adding them to soups at first.

See pages 44-45 for pictures and a listing of a variety of vegetables.

## FRUITS

Fruits are a good source of vitamins, especially vitamins A and C, minerals, natural sugars, fiber, and water.[1]

Fresh fruits should be eaten ripe, since their simple sugars are then more easily digested and assimilated. Try to use fruits that are in season.

Dried fruits contain "food energy", or calories, fiber, minerals, and some vitamins. Be sure your dried fruits are "unsulfured", which means that the toxic chemical, sulfur dioxide, has not been added. (See p.321, "unsulfured" in the Glossary.)

For many people, oranges and grapefruit are too acidic, and should be limited.

See page 46 for pictures and a listing of many of the most common fruits.

## SWEETENERS

raw honey                    barley malt
unsulphured molasses         pure maple syrup
rice bran syrup              pure fruit juices
unsweetened carob powder
unsulfured dried fruit

A note on honey vs. sugar: Although the body reacts to honey as sugar, raw honey has some nutrients and antibiotic properties that sugar does not have. Therefore, honey gives the body something in return, while sugar does nothing but cause depletion and stress.

Molasses and maple syrup, although "natural" sugars, are extremely concentrated.

Don't over-do your use of any of these natural sweeteners.

## SEASONINGS

cayenne pepper (Add after cooking to preserve the vitamin C and niacin.)
sea salt contains 75% sodium as well as
   other minerals, and is therefore more
   balanced and less stressful than common
   table salt, which is pure sodium
   chloride. However, limit all salts.
gomasio (sea salt & roasted sesame seeds)
soy sauce
apple cider vinegar (unpasteurized, if
   possible)
pure vanilla, orange or almond extract
dried vegetable powders and powdered dulse
   or kelp, which are powdered seaweeds
herbs and spices:

| | | | |
|---|---|---|---|
| allspice | comfrey | mustard | dill |
| oregano | caraway | nutmeg | basil |
| bay leaves | parsley | oregano | sage |
| coriander | garlic | cloves | mint |
| chili powder | cinnamon | ginger | thyme |
| tarragon | marjoram | chives | cumin |

-43-

# VEGETABLES

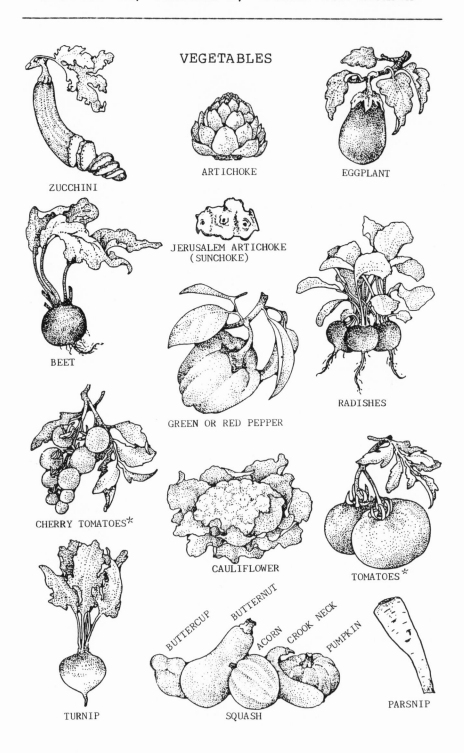

ZUCCHINI

ARTICHOKE

EGGPLANT

JERUSALEM ARTICHOKE
(SUNCHOKE)

BEET

RADISHES

GREEN OR RED PEPPER

CHERRY TOMATOES*

CAULIFLOWER

TOMATOES*

TURNIP

BUTTERCUP  BUTTERNUT  ACORN  CROOK NECK  PUMPKIN

SQUASH

PARSNIP

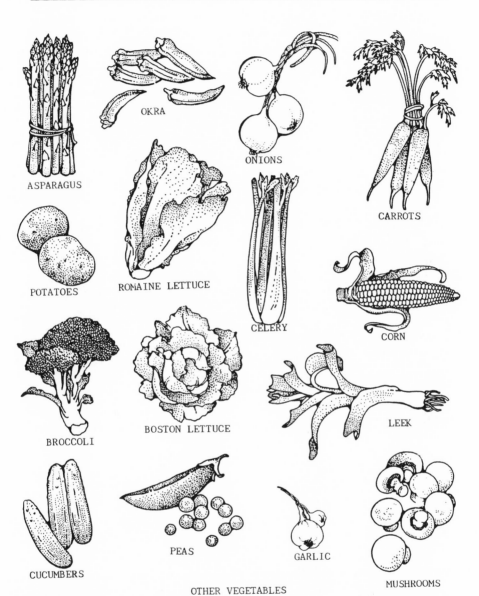

ASPARAGUS

OKRA

ONIONS

CARROTS

POTATOES

ROMAINE LETTUCE

CELERY

CORN

BROCCOLI

BOSTON LETTUCE

LEEK

CUCUMBERS

PEAS

GARLIC

MUSHROOMS

OTHER VEGETABLES

| | | | |
|---|---|---|---|
| RED CABBAGE | YAM | SNOW PEAS | WATERCHESTNUT |
| WHITE CABBAGE | SWEET POTATO | LIMA BEANS | GREEN STRING BEAN |
| CHINESE CABBAGE | DAIKON RADISH | SCALLIONS | YELLOW STRING BEAN |

LEAFY GREENS: WATERCRESS, PARSLEY, BASIL, MINT, CARROT TOPS, BEET GREENS, TURNIP GREENS, DANDELION GREENS, MUSTARD GREENS, KALE, SWISS CHARD, SPINACH, SORREL, ENDIVE, COMFREY, ESCAROLE, CHICKORY, RUGALA.

EDIBLE SEA VEGETABLES: KOMBU, HIJIKI, DULSE, ARAME, WAKAME, KANTEN, KELP

* Note: Although tomatoes are actually a fruit, they are usually eaten as if a vegetable.

# FRUITS

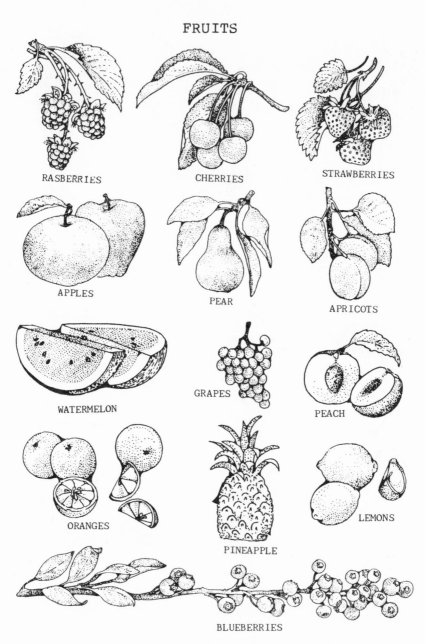

RASBERRIES CHERRIES STRAWBERRIES

APPLES PEAR APRICOTS

WATERMELON GRAPES PEACH

ORANGES PINEAPPLE LEMONS

BLUEBERRIES

OTHER FRUITS

| PAPAYA | MANGO | RAISIN | PRUNE | KIWI |
| BANANA | CURRANT | FIG | PERSIMMON | AVOCADO |

CHAPTER 2

AVOIDING STRESSFUL FOODS

Foods which contribute to mental and physical deterioration are those foods which are farthest from their natural state. They have been processed, refined, adulterated with chemicals, sugar or salt, over-cooked, fried, or are rancid.

Processed foods harm the body in several ways:
(1)They have no nutrients so they give nothing to the body; or,
(2) They are toxic or stressful, because of their additives, or manner of processing or cooking.
(3) They demand energy and nutrients to digest and assimilate;
(4) They fill you up, replacing foods which do nourish you. This is one reason "junk" foods encourage weight gain and im-balance of the entire metabolism.
(5) Because of the above reasons, they contribute to chronic disease, such as dia-betes, heart disease, etc.

Learn to read labels. Keep in your pocket a list of the most common food additives and their level of toxicity. Not all additives are toxic. For a guide in distinguishing between which are toxic and which are not, refer to the Appendix for a list of additives most commonly used in packaged foods.

In addition to toxic additives, processed foods are heavily dosed with sugar or salt. Americans consume 30-40 Tablespoons of sugar per day, and 10 times more salt than is needed.¹·The major portion of the sugar and salt consumed is in processed foods, not in that which is added by the consumer to a meal. If you feel you eat very little salt or sugar, but still eat processed foods, read labels, and refer to the lists of "Hidden Sugars" and "Hidden Salt" in Foods, pp.306 and 307. You may be in for a surprise.

Keep in mind that ingredients are listed in order of weight - the highest amount listed first. For example, if sugar is listed first, there is more sugar than any other ingredient. Also remember that there are many types of sugar. See p.49.

In many cases the ingredients do not have to be listed and there are "hidden" sugars and other chemicals. Whenever possible, use fresh foods rather than packaged.

In cases where there is a risk of fresh fruits and vegetables being contaminated by pesticides and preservatives, it helps to wash them in a particular way. Refer to "Kitchen Hints".

Ask for only the best and purest foods in your life. If you refuse to buy processed foods, there will eventually be a change in the market place. It's an investment in your good health, and you deserve it!

******** STRESSFUL FOODS TO AVOID ********

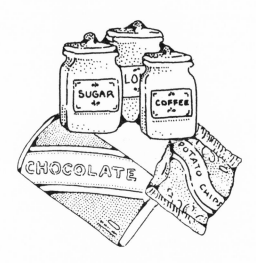

SUGGESTION: LEARN TO BE A GOOD LABEL READER

## "FOODS" LACED WITH SUGAR OR SALT.

Sugar comes in many forms - white, brown, turbinado (which is white sugar with molasses added), glucose, fructose, sucrose, corn syrup, dextrose, nutri-sweet, etc. Any refined sweetener is devoid of nutritive value and creates tremendous stress on the entire body.

Sugar contributes to tooth decay and gum disease, acne, obesity, hypoglycemia, diabetes, arthritis, heart disease, alcoholism, drug addiction, schizophrenia, nervous and behavioral disorders, - in general, to poor digestion, assimilation and elimination, thus increasing susceptibility to all disease.[2]

Many packaged and canned foods contain sugar. Read labels, and be aware of "hidden" sugars in foods. Refer to the "Hidden Sugars" chart, p.306 in the Appendix.

Salt affects the water balance in the body's cells, can be detrimental to the circulatory system, and lead to potassium deficiency and is known to be a contributory factor in digestive disorders, kidney disease, nervous disorders, hypertension, cancer and heart ailment.[3]

Refer to the Appendix, p.307, for a list of hidden salt in processed food.

"FOODS" WITH TOXIC ADDITIVES, such as MSG, BHA, BHT, sodium nitrate and nitrite, artificial color and flavor, etc. should be avoided. See "Common Food Additives" in the Appendix. These additives are extremely stressful to the body, contributing to numerous disorders including cancer, schizophrenia and hyperactivity. A difficult child may be a very sick child - a product of adulterated food.[1]

Foods that frequently contain toxic additives are the following:[2]

* Bacon, frankfurters, sausage, liverwurst, pork, bologna, salami, tongue, corned beef, pastrami, smoked fish, gefilte fish, packaged seafood, canned ham.

* Canned soups, soup mixes, canned vegetables, canned sauces, canned tomato paste, bouillon cubes.

* Bottled salad dressings, vegetable shortenings, jams, jellies, mayonnaise, ketchup, meat tenderizers.

* Processed cheeses, frozen pizzas, cheese spreads, butter, margarine.

* Dry roasted nuts, red pistachio nuts.

* Baby formulas.

* Packaged cakes and cake mixes, packaged cookies, crackers, pies, doughnuts, pretzels, pastry icings and fillings, jello, puddings, gelatin, frozen desserts, ice cream, ice milk, whipped toppings, sugar substitutes, chewing gum.

Colas, soft drinks, chocolate milk, evaporated milk, punches, powders, beer, cocoa, instant teas.

Many of the above listed foods can be purchased in the health food store without toxic additives. However, be sure to read labels even in the health food store, and work toward preparing foods as fresh and as home made as possible.

PROCESSED AND REFINED FLOURS, GRAINS CEREALS AND NOODLES, such as white flour, white rice, etc. These "foods" are mostly starch, with almost all essential nutrients (vitamins E, B, and other vitamins and minerals, protein, and fiber) removed.[1] They require work and energy to metabolize while giving you no nutrients in return, and they fill you up so that you have no room for the foods that do support you.[2]

"Enriched" grains contain only a few synthetic vitamins, replacing about 25 nutrients removed in processing.[3] Refined products often contain sugar, salt, stabilizers, bleach and other potentially toxic additives.[4]

Use of these foods increases susceptibility to disease. They contribute to obesity, disorders of digestion, metabolism and elimination, to vitamin and mineral deficiency diseases, nervous and other disorders. Evidence shows that lack of fiber in the diet may be a major contributory factor in the rise of colon and other forms of cancer, in hemmorhoids, varicose veins, appendicitis, heart disease, diabetes, and other chronic disorders.[5]

MEATS INJECTED WITH HORMONES, ANTI-BIOTICS, TRANQUILIZERS, ARSENIC, OR OTHER CHEMICALS, and raised on chemical feed! Hormones in the meats may contribute to hormonal imbalances in humans, to sterility and cancer. Our excessive consumption of anti-biotics, including in our meats, has given rise to a strain of antibiotic resistant bacteria. This may seriously undermine the effectuality of antibiotics in medicine.

It is not necessary to avoid meat altogether. However, there are essentially 4 categories of cautionary considerations when choosing your meat, other than cost, digesti-bility and other factors one considers when choosing whether or not to eat meat at all, which is a subject beyond the scope of this Handbook. The following are factors to consider once you have made the decision to include meat in your diet:

(1) The level of adulteration. Try to avoid meat from animals that are injected with hormones and antibiotics, and are fed chemical feed. Keep in mind that it is in the liver, skin and fatty portions of the meat that the toxins are particularly concentrat-ed.[2] Also avoid luncheon meats and bacon packaged with nitrates, possible carcinogens.

Whenever possible, get organic meat; that is, meat from animals that have not been injected, and have been raised free-range on their natural feed. Sometimes health food stores and fine meat markets carry organic meat and liver, and hot dogs and bacon with-out nitrates. Occasionally kosher meat is organic, and lamb is usually not injected.

(2) The level of "natural" contamina-tion. Pork often contains parasites which are extremely resistent to high heat and prolong-ed cooking. Sometimes raw fish contains para-sites, and shell fish can be contaminated. Choose fish that is preferably in season and from a reputable store or restaurant.

(3) The fat in meat may contribute to heart disease. Choose lean meat. Cut off any fatty portions of meats, and remove the skins

(4) The method of cooking. Avoid fried and smoked meats. High heats cause cancer-causing substances in these fats.

All of these "avoids" concerning meat may sound overwhelming. Again, work with the good, better, best guide. Probably chicken, fish or lamb are best. Get the best meat that is available. Then enjoy it. If you are primarily eating the high fiber, high nutrient foods listed in Chapter 1, your body should be able to balance out the effects of toxins and fat in the meat.

HIGH HEATED, RANCID, HYDROGENATED AND PROCESSED OILS. Oils heated to high temperatures, particularly beyond 250°, become difficult to digest,[1] irritate the gastro-intestinal lining, contribute to heart disease, and are converted to toxic, cancer causing substances.[2]

When foods are cooked in high-heated oils, such as in high heat frying, barbecuing and smoking, cancer-causing substances are formed in the foods,[3] and polyunsaturated oils are converted to toxins which prevent the utilization of other dietary oils. In cooking with oils, cook on low heats. Use olive oil or butter, which are least affected by high heat. Make your own potato chips and french fries on low heats.

Heating oils also results in a loss of lecithin and many minerals and vitamins, including vitamin E which, in addition to being a vitamin we need for good health, prevents the oil from becoming rancid.[4]

Oils and oil-based foods, such as nuts and seeds, nut butters and wheat germ become rancid at room temperature. Always keep them in the refrigerator or freezer.

Most commercially processed oils are subjected to high heats, bleaching and deodorizing, and contain toxic or questionable chemicals, such as BHA and BHT.[5]

When oils are hydrogenated, or artificially hardened, to produce margarine or shortenings, many vitamins, minerals and essential fatty acids are lost. In addition, the structure of the fat molecule is altered in such a way that it becomes difficult to utilize. Recent evidence suggests that hydrogenated fats may contribute to heart disease.[6]

In summary, when using oils, use oils which have been processed and heated as little as possible. These are the "cold - pressed oils". Remember to cook on low heats. (See "Foods to Enjoy - Oils", p.41.)

OILS WHICH ARE DIFFICULT TO DIGEST, such as coconut, palm, cottonseed, safflower, peanut, corn. These oils put tremendous strain on the liver. (Soy oil is normally one of the better oils nutritionally. Use it in moderation, however as it is a common allergen and can contribute to congestion.)[1]

OVERCONSUMPTION OF ALCOHOL encourages birth defects, complications of pregnancy, and hypoglycemia, a precursor to diabetes. It can destroy brain cells, harm blood vessels, the heart, nerves and other organs.

Alcohol depletes the body of nutrients. It requires vitamins, minerals and enzymes to be detoxified. It depresses the appetite, and interferes with digestion and assimilation.[1]

As a "transition" alcohol, some people more easily tolerate pure vodka with tomato juice and a dash of cayenne pepper. Use less vodka each time, and more tomato juice and cayenne. Cayenne contains calcium, Vitamin C and niacin to give you extra support in overcoming the effects of the alcohol.

Eating food, especially protein and raw vegetables, while drinking alcohol also helps balance the negative effects of the alcohol.


PASTEURIZED, HOMOGENIZED MILK AND ITS PRODUCTS , especially cow's milk, are common allergens, encouraging gastro-intestinal disorders, asthma, hay fever, arthritis and other chronic disease, as well as hyper-activity and other behavioral problems. For many people, they are extremely mucous forming, and are generally congesting.[1]

Heating proteins, such as in pasteurizing milk, decreases its digestibility. Some research suggests that homogenized milk may contribute to heart disease.[2]

Commercial milk often contains hormones, antibiotics, radioactive isotopes, pesticides and other pollutants.[3]

See "Foods to Enjoy- Dairy", p.40, for dairy products that are less stressful.


CAFFEINE AND TANNIN CONTAINING BEVERAGES SUCH AS COFFEE, BLACK TEAS AND COLAS. Caffeine is over-stimulating to the heart and can aggrevate stomach ulcers,[1] nervousness, headaches, skin,[2] intestinal and other disorders.[3] It also interferes with the use of iron and certain vitamins, and creates B deficiencies, contributing to stress.[4]

Tannin can damage the liver and mucous membrane of the mouth and digestive tract, interfering with digestion and elimination.[5]


CHOCOLATE is high in fat, and calories and sugar, since its natural bitter taste requires the addition of sugar.[1] It has theo-bromine and caffeine, which are excessively stimulating to the heart,[2] and has oxalic acid which inhibits the metabolism of calcium.[3]

Chocolate is usually an allergen, and contributes to skin problems, constipation, breathing and digestive difficulties, cystic breast disease, herpes, depressive mood swings and other disorders.[4]

ALLERGENS are foods which can in certain cases trigger allergy symptoms, such as headaches, insomnia, abdominal distress, poor concentration and coordination, anxiety, dizziness, fatique, asthma, hyperactivity and other behavior problems, mood swings with no apparent cause, sudden anger, runny nose, dark circles under the eyes, and an excessive craving for the allergen.

It is as if one is "addicted" to the allergen. Eating it makes one feel better, since it postpones the withdrawal symptoms, but ultimately perpetuates the addiction syndrome, contributing to further weakness.[1]

The most common food allergens are sugar, artificial food colors, cow's milk, wheat, corn, rye, barley, oats, chocolate, eggs, coffee, cola, peanuts, walnuts, pecans, citrus, beef, pork, bananas, white potatoes, tomatoes, cinnamon, fish, shrimp, onion, garlic, yeast, snap beans and dried peas.

To avoid eating a food allergen is helpful, but it is more important to find out why the body is rejecting the food. Allergic reactions can be caused by lack of digestive enzymes, malnourishment, weak adrenal and digestive function, and over all toxicity. A latent food allergy can manifest from eating too much of one food too often. This is one reason it is so important to vary your foods.[2]

If you suspect a food allergy, avoid it for 5-7 days, then eat it first thing in the morning and see how you respond. There are various other tests, including blood tests, and taking your pulse after eating, which can help you identify the allergens.[3] Consult your nutrition consultant or physician.

CHAPTER 3


LOW STRESS CHANGE


Although there are generally foods which support good health (the "Foods to Enjoy") and foods which encourage ill health (the "Foods to Avoid"), diets vary with each person and with different points in each person's life. There is no one target diet appropriate for everyone at all times. We are always more or less in a state of transition.

Following is a "Transition Chart" which is a simplification, but a helpful guide in grasping an over-all picture of which foods are never supportive at any time; which foods are sometimes necessary; and which foods are supportive at any point. (Naturally, there are always exceptions, such as with food sensitivities.)

As you can see, Column (1) corresponds to the "Foods to Avoid" listed in the previous chapter, while Columns (2) and (3) correspond to the "Foods to Enjoy" list.

Column (1), "Foods to Avoid", are stressful to everyone and should be given up as soon as possible.

Column (2), "Acceptable Foods", may be an important part of your health regime, or may be stressful, depending on your particular reaction. Some of these foods may be part of your menus temporarily, and some may be a permanent part of your diet.

Column (3), "Vital Foods", generally support health and vitality.

Most people find the best diet for them combines foods in Columns (2) and (3). They continuously add and subtract foods from Column (2), as their needs change, while in-including most foods from Column (3).

Following is a visual representation of the usual progression of a transition:

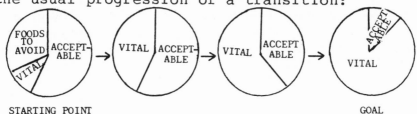

STARTING POINT                                    GOAL

The circle represents your total diet at one time. You should eliminate the "Foods to Avoid" as soon as possible, then gradually cut down on the "Acceptable" foods, but not eliminate them altogether. Again, certain "Acceptable" foods may be as supportive for you as the "Vital" foods. "Vital" foods Only should not necessarily be a goal. The ratio of "Acceptable" foods to "Vital" foods is an individual decision. However, your diet should primarily consist of "Vital" foods.

-58-

## TRANSITION CHART

| | FOODS TO AVOID | FOODS TO ENJOY | |
|---|---|---|---|
| | | Acceptable Foods | Vital Foods |
| | Eliminate Immediately | Experiment with These | Primarily Use These |
| PROTEINS | Meats with additives, such as luncheon meat packed with nitrites (bologna, salami, etc)<br>Processed cheese<br>Battery eggs*<br>Battery chicken*<br>Meat with hormones,etc.<br>Pork; Veal<br>Pasteurized, homogenized cow's milk<br>Yogurt with sugar, and toxic additives<br>*Battery:Raised in small coops, injected with antibiotics, etc. | Meat without additives, hormones,antibiotics, etc., raised free-range on organic feed<br>Deep ocean or pure-lake fish<br>Certified Raw Milk<br>Raw cheese<br>Yogurt without toxic additives<br>Raw soured milk<br>Cultured buttermilk<br>Cottage cheese without toxic additives<br>Dry milk powder without toxic additives | Sprouts<br>Fresh, raw nuts and seeds: flax, chia, pumpkin, sunflower, sesame, almond, pecan, brazil, walnut, filbert, etc.<br>Nut butters<br>Nut milks<br>Organic Eggs |
| CARBOHYDRATES | Sugar: white, brown, turbinado, sucrose, glucose, corn syrup, fructose, etc.<br>Chocolate<br>Processed carbohydrate such as white flour and white flour products<br>White rice<br>Anything packaged or canned with sugar, salt or toxic additives<br>Processed noodles<br>Ice cream with sugar and toxic additives | Raw honey; unsulphured molasses; barley malt; pure maple syrup<br>Carob<br>Whole Grain Bread<br>Whole Grain Noodles<br>Pure ice cream made without toxic additives or sugar | Vegetables:squash, carrots, celery, tomatoes, beets, cabbage, broccoli, cauliflower, leeks, turnips, radish, lettuce, etc.<br>Fruit: apple,grape, bananas, papayas, pineapple, peach, melon, etc.<br>Sea Vegetables<br>Whole Grains:brown rice, millet, rye, barley, etc.<br>Beans:lentils, soy beans, split peas, black beans, etc. |
| LIPIDS | Oils that are rancid or difficult to digest (see "Foods to Avoid")<br>Rancid animal fats, such as lard, bacon drippings, etc.<br>Anything deep-fat fried<br>Artificially hardened fats, such as margarine and shortenings | Oils which are un-rancid and not over-heated<br>Unsalted non-raw butter | Raw, cold-pressed oils: olive, sunflower, sesame, flax, almond, walnut, avocado, soy<br>Raw, unsalted butter<br>Avocado<br>Fresh, raw nuts and seeds |
| OTHER | Coffee, tannic-acid teas; excess alcohol<br>Common Table Salt<br>Any commercial condiments with sugar, salt or toxic additives<br>Commercial soft drink and commercial ice cream made with toxic additives and sugar | Pure grain coffee substitutes<br>Not-more-than 1 glass a day of non-chemicalized wine or beer<br>Aluminum-free baking powder<br>Soft drinks made without chemicals,sugar or toxic additives<br>Soy sauce without toxic additives<br>Potassium balanced salt; Sea salt<br>Vegetable salt and kelp | Herb teas and seasonings<br>Organic apple cider vinegar<br>Home-made condiments without salt or sugar<br>Freshly juiced vegetables and fruits.<br>Fresh fruit ice cream<br>Spring water |

If the "Foods to Avoid" comprise a major part of your diet, and you are in a state of shock at the prospect of eliminating them immediately, don't be discouraged. "Immediately" really means as soon as possible, but it may take you a while to eliminate them altogether. There will probably be times when it is relatively easy for you to avoid them. Then, many times you will "slip" because of the social situation you are in, or because of old habits and cravings for the taste or familiarity for the food. Keep working at it. Eventually you will loose your taste for them. (Honest! Even I did.) At that point you simply won't want or need to eat them.

Remember that there are many delicious foods which will more than replace these non-foods, and which will make your transition easier and more enjoyable than you can imagine. It is simply a matter of education, experimentation and discovery.

Your increased health and vitality will also give you the encouragement to take the next steps.

---

CHAPTER 4


PRACTICAL TIPS FOR A SMOOTH TRANSITION
CONVERTING AND SUPPLEMENTING RECIPES


Psychologically as well as physically it is easier to adapt to a new diet if you begin with recipes to which you are accustomed, but with health changes.

You can convert old recipes, substituting healthful ingredients for stressful ones, such as whole wheat flour for white flour, and you can supplement old recipes with ingredients which add flavor and a nutritional boost.

An added bonus for converting and supplementing recipes: You will be happily surprised at how much more delicious your recipes will be!

CONVERT YOUR RECIPES

In converting recipes, you can totally replace processed ingredients (such as sugar, white flour, white rice, white noodles) with more pure sweeteners and whole grain ingredients, following the simple guidelines on the next few pages.

You can also add the whole grain ingredients gradually, using a mixture of processed and whole grain until you and your family are accustomed to the new color and taste. For example, mix brown and white rice together, whole wheat and white flour, whole grain and white noodles.


Following are some guidelines for converting your recipes.

You will note that I have included conversion tips for whole wheat flour to other flours, and for eggs to other ingredients. Although whole wheat and eggs are normally good foods, many people are allergic to wheat and eggs, as well as dairy, and need substitutes.

******** CONVERTING YOUR RECIPES ********

SUGAR TO HONEY

In Beverages: to taste

In Baking:
    Use 1/2 to 3/4 cup honey for 1 cup sugar, depending on how sweet you want it (usually 1/2).
    Reduce the amount of liquid in the recipe 1/4 cup for each cup of honey used. For example, if 1/2 cup of honey is used, reduce the liquid by 2 Tablespoons.
    In cakes which call for no liquid, where crispness is important, add 4 Tablespoons additional flour for every 1 cup honey.
    Lower the oven temperature by about 25° since honey browns more quickly than sugar.
    To make it easier to measure the honey without having it stick to the measuring cup, lightly oil the cup first. Or, if the recipe calls for oil, measure the oil first.
    If you wish to liquify honey, for easier measuring and blending, gently warm it (See "Natural Food Kitchen Hints" in "Appendix".)


SUGAR TO MOLASSES

In Beverages: to taste

In Baking:
    Usually, molasses, rather than honey, is used in place of brown sugar.
    Use 1/2 to 3/4 c. molasses in place of brown sugar.
    Reduce the amount of liquid in the recipe by 1/4 cup for each cup of molasses.

Note: When a recipe calls for 1 cup white sugar and 1 cup brown sugar, use 3/4 cup honey and 1/4 cup molasses.


SALT TO SOY SAUCE, SUCH AS TAMARI, OR TO POWDERED SEAWEED, SUCH AS KELP OR DULSE POWDER, OR TO SALT-FREE VEGETABLE "SALT"

    To taste. Begin with small amounts. Keep in mind that kelp and soy sauce will turn the food a darker color, and that kelp has a "seaweed" taste. If you are allergic to wheat, make sure your soy sauce is wheat-free.
    As a very first step, you may want to use sea salt in place of common table salt. Use it to taste. Sea salt has no chemicals added to it to make it flow freely, and has been dried naturally in the sun.

CHOCOLATE TO CAROB

In recipes that call for solid chocolate, use 3 Tablespoons carob powder plus 2 Tablespoons water or nut milk (See Recipes, "Nut Milk".) to one square of chocolate. (One square is usually equal to one ounce.)
Be sure to use carob powder that has no added sugar. There is also roasted and unroasted carob powder. Most people prefer the roasted.
Carob dissolves better in oil than in water.
To help get rid of the raw taste of carob, mix it with hot liquid.
Ground filbert nuts, vanilla extract and a little molasses helps to give carob more of a "chocolate" taste. However, carob can be delicious in its own right. Don't expect it to taste just like chocolate, and you won't be disappointed.

WHITE FLOUR TO WHOLE WHEAT FLOUR

In general, remove 2 Tablespoons of whole wheat flour for every 1 cup of white flour, particularly with sifted white flour.
For example, 2 cups sifted white flour equals 1 3/4 cups sifted whole wheat flour. And, 2 cups unsifted white flour equals 2 cups sifted whole wheat flour.
If you are using coarse ground wheat, remove 2 Tablespoons whole wheat flour for every one cup of white flour. Omit sifting. Just stir lightly.
Whole wheat pastry flour is lighter, and better suited for cakes and cookies than whole wheat flour. Use the same proportions as for whole wheat.

WHOLE WHEAT FLOUR TO OTHER FLOURS

Although whole wheat is a nutritious grain, many people have wheat allergies.
For 1 cup of wheat use any of the following:
        1 1/4 c. rye flour
        1/2 c. rye flour + 1/2 c. potato flour
        2/3 c. rye flour + 1/3 c. cooked potato
        1 c. millet flour
        1/2 c. millet flour and 1/2 c. cooked potato
        (either white or sweet, depending on the
        taste you want)
        1/4 c. ground nuts and/or seeds + 3/4 c.
          cooked potato
        3/4 c. cooked potato + 2 Tbl. soy flour
        1 c. corn flour
        7/8 c. rice flour
        1/2 c. rice flour + 1/2 c. oat flour

## NOTES ON CONVERTING WHOLE WHEAT TO OTHER FLOURS:

Millet flour has a "bite" to it so it is best in recipes with an ingredient which overpowers the "bite" such as in a spice cake or a banana bread (See "Breads").

If you use potato flour or cooked potato, you may need to increase the liquid amount. If you use cooked potato, measure by quickly grinding it in the blender. Blend the cooked potato with the liquid and spices, then add to the dry ingredients. Millet flour or ground nuts work well with cooked potato.

Soy flour is difficult to digest and has a strong, slightly unpleasant taste, so it is best not to use more than 2 Tbl. to a cup, or 1/8 of your total flour volumn.
Since soy is high in protein and fat, it causes heavy browning of the crust. Therefore, if you use a large amount of soy flour, reduce the oven temperature by 25°.
Since soy flour is high in fat, it should be mixed with the wet ingredients rather than the dry.
Soy four acts as a preservative. Breads made with it stay fresh longer.
A small amount of soy flour in your breads will make them a more complete protein. (See "Protein Combining".)

Rice flour is quite heavy, so it is best mixed with another, lighter flour. In addition, beating the egg whites till they from soft peaks, and folding them into the batter, will make the cake, bread, muffins, etc. lighter in texture.

## WHITE RICE TO BROWN RICE

Use the same amounts, but plan on more cooking time, depending on the method used. (See "Grains".)

## MILK TO "NUT MILK" (See "Beverages")

Nut Milk is a milky looking liquid made by blending ground nuts and/or seeds, or nut butter, with water. (See "Beverages".) Nut milk can be used in place of milk in any recipe and will add the taste of the nut or seed.
"Almond Milk", which has a delicious, mild flavor, is particularly good in place of milk.
Use the same amounts of nut milk as you would cow's milk.
Raw goat milk is often well tolerated in place of cow's milk. However, it is difficult to find and, although some goat milk is delicious, especially when fresh, the taste is often disliked.

EGGS TO OTHER INGREDIENTS

For one egg use any of the following:

    1 teaspoon arrowroot flour
    1 teaspoon yam flour
    1 teaspoon sweet rice flour

Or, for baking, use 1 Tablespoon lecithin for 1 egg. Blend it fast with an oil included in the recipe. Then, if the recipe calls for a sweetener, blend with that.
Or, to cold water add 1 cup ground flaxseed. Bring to a boil, stirring constantly. Boil for 3 minutes. Let cool, then place in the refrigerator in a closed jar. Whenever your recipe calls for 1 beaten egg, substitute 1 Tablespoon of the above mixture.
Or, Dissolve 1 package unflavored gelatin in hot water. 2 to 3 Tablespoons of that is good in cheesecakes and pies.
Or, Soak 1/2 pound apricots in 2 cups water overnight. The next morning, beat or blend them. Add water, if needed. Strain them and store in the refrigerator. Every time your recipe calls for beaten eggs, take a generous Tablespoon of this and blend with your recipe.

ANIMAL FATS, LARD, SHORTENING TO BUTTER

    Use 1 cup butter in place of any of the following:

    2 cups commercial shortening
    1 cup margarine
    4/5 cup bacon fat (clarified)
    3/4 cup chicken fat
    7/8 cup cottonseed, corn, nut oil
    7/8 cup lard
    4/5 to 7/8 cup drippings

Note that sesame butter or tahini can be used as a shortening for bread or cookies in place of butter or other fat.

## SUPPLEMENTING YOUR RECIPES

Another tip for making your transition smooth, and your recipes more delicious and power-packed, is to supplement them with ingredients which add nourishment.

## ***** SUPPLEMENTS TO ENRICH YOUR MEALS *****

### SUPPLEMENT YOUR MEALS WITH NOURISHMENT

| SUPPLEMENT | SPECIAL NUTRIENT | ADD IT TO |
|---|---|---|
| Bran (wheat or rice) | Fiber | Breads, cakes, cookies, cereals, beverages and blender drinks, loaves, casseroles, etc. |
| Cayenne pepper | Vitamin C; calcium | Add after cooking to vegetable juice, soups, steamed vegetables, grains, sauces, dressings, etc. |
| Kelp or dulse powder | Iodine and other minerals | Use whenever you would use salt, but would not mind a light sea-weed taste. |
| Molasses (unsulphured) | potassium, iron, trace minerals | Add to water as a beverage; in blender drinks, cereals, cookies, etc. (Don't overdo.) |
| Nutritional Yeast* | Vitamin B complex | Beverages, blender drinks, bread, cookies, soups, loaves and casseroles, burgers, etc. |
| Nuts & Seeds whole, ground, as milks | Protein and many vitamins and minerals | casseroles, loaves, burgers, cereals, breads, beverages and blender drinks, sauces, dressings, snacks, on salads and desserts. |
| Parsley | Vitamin A & C; iron and other minerals | Juices, soups, dressings, sauces, salads, vegetables, loaves, burgers, grains, beans, meats, etc. |
| Rice polishings | Silicon and Vitamin B | Beverages, blender drinks, bread, cookies, soups, loaves, burgers, casseroles, sauces, etc. |
| Soy powder | Protein; B vitamins | Beverages and blender drinks, soups, casseroles, loaves, bread, cookies, etc. (Don't overdo. It's hard to digest.) |
| Sprouts | Enzymes, protein, vitamins A, C and many other vitamins and minerals and fiber | salads, sandwiches, sauces, dressings, soups, omelettes, loaves, etc. Add last to hot things. Don't cook, if possible, as cooking kills many of the nutrients. |
| Wheat germ* (vacuum packed) | B vitamins, Vitamin E, protein, potassium and phosphorus | Beverages and blender drinks, breads, cookies, cakes, cereals, loaves and casseroles, burgers, on salads or desserts. |

* Except in cases of allergies to yeast or wheat.

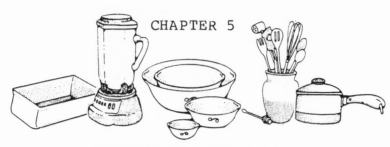

CHAPTER 5

EQUIPMENT & UTENSILS

    The equipment and utensils used in the preparation of foods can save time, and can help you prepare food that is packed with nutrition.

    The following pages contain pictures, and a listing of the most basic equipment and utensils. Some of them can be used in the following ways:

    <u>FLAME TAMER</u> is extremely helpful for low-heat cooking. It is simply a wire frame or fire-proof pad designed to buffer the heat between the stove top and the pot. If you cannot locate one in a store, make your own with a wire or wire hanger.

    <u>BLENDER</u> is wonderful for making "smoothies", "green drinks", blended salads, nut milks, grain water, creamy cereals, sauces, dips, dressings, fruit ice creams, soups, etc. See "Recipes". Most people find that a simple blender with 4 speeds is sufficient.

    <u>JUICER</u> extracts juice from fruits or vegetables. There are various types of juicers. The "press type" is preferable for best preserving food nutrients, although other kinds may be simpler to use. Some types also double for mashing frozen fruits into ice creams, or sprouted grains into breads.

GRATER grates raw vegetables such as carrots, beets, sweet potatoes, etc. for making salads, loaves, etc.

NUT-SEED GRINDER grinds nuts and seeds for nut milks, nut/seed loaves or patties, or to add to breads, salads, cereals, etc. It also grinds grains or beans as flour for cereals, breads, etc.

STEAMER is for steaming vegetables, heating cooked grains or noodles, etc.

GARLIC PRESS is for mincing garlic.

TIMER helps prevent over-cooked food.

VEGETABLE BRUSH is handy for scrubbing skins of vegetables that should be eaten with skins (when not heavily sprayed with pesticides) such as carrots, potatoes, Jerusalem artichokes (sunchokes).


PLEASE NOTE:
Do not cook with aluminum or copper cookware as there is some evidence that they leach toxic levels of metal into the food and pull "life energy" from the food. High levels of aluminum have been shown to impair the nervous system, contributing to liver and kidney failure and Alzheimer's Disease.[1.]
Stainless steel, pyrex, iron, black steel or enamel is best.
If you use black steel, turn the oven down 10° since it absorbs and holds heat more than other cook ware.
If you use enamel, be sure it is not chipped.

# EQUIPMENT
# &
# UTENSILS

blender

wok

juicer

cutting board

toaster oven

food processor

loaf pans

mixing bowls

casserole pan

sauce pans

double boiler

frying pans
(small & large)

grater/shredder

colander

steamer

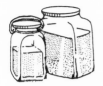
glass jars
(for storing food)

grinder (hand and/or electric)

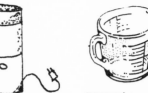
measuring cup

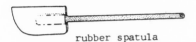
rubber spatula

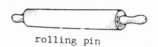
rolling pin

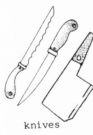
pot holders

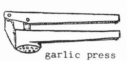
garlic press

measuring spoons

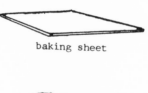
baking sheet

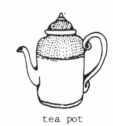
tea pot

knives

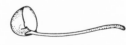
strainer

soup ladle

OTHER UTENSILS

| | | |
|---|---|---|
| sprouting equipment (glass jar, cheese cloth, rubber band) | timer | water filter |
| | wire whisk | kitchen shears |
| | spatula | vegetable brush |
| spoons(stainless & wooden) | tea kettle | wooden salad bowl |
| asbestos pad or flame tamer | crock pot | |

-71-

CHAPTER 6

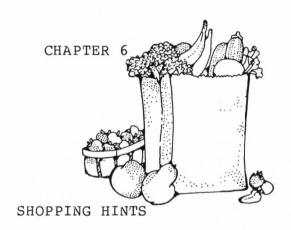

SHOPPING HINTS

Easy shopping and a knowledge of which staples to have on hand adds to stress-free food preparation. Here are some hints:

(1) Buy grain, flour, beans and peas and nuts and seeds in bulk. Put grains, flour and nuts and seeds in covered glass or porcelain jars in the refrigerator to keep them fresh. (Nuts and seeds keep even better in the freezer.) (See "Kitchen Hints", pp. 299-301, for other storage hints.)
(2) When you buy ingredients for a meal, you may want to buy extra, to prepare something for the next day.
(3) Try to buy perishable foods as close to a meal as possible.
(4) Note staples necessary for this meal that may be low.
(5) Note foods already on hand.

STAPLES

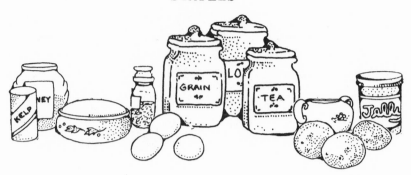

These are foods which keep well, which you can have on hand all the time. Please be sure they are as unadulterated as possible. See "Availability Chart", p.13 for where you can buy these staples.

Staples can be divided into three categories:

A. Those which store over a longer period of time. These can be purchased once a month, or less.

B. Those which keep fairly well. These can be purchased once a week.

C. The more perishable foods, such as certain fruits and vegetables, which may need to be purchased every couple of days. These are not included on this list.

## GROUP A - PURCHASE ONCE A MONTH, OR LESS

BEVERAGES...... grain coffee substitutes
herb teas
pure bottled juices
spring or distilled water.
CEREALS*....... home-made granola or good
quality store bought.
SEASONINGS..... herbs and spices; herb and
vegetable salt substitutes
apple cider vinegar*;
soy sauce; kelp powder
onions, garlic.
CRACKERS....... rice, rye and/or wheat.

---

```
DRIED BEANS....  aduki, garbanzo, kidney,
                 lentil, split pea, mung
                 (for cooking & sprouting)
DRIED FRUIT....  (unsulfured) raisins,
                 dates, figs, etc.
EXTRACTS.......  pure vanilla,orange,almond
FLOUR*.........  whole grain rye, wheat,
                 pastry wheat, millet, etc.
GRAINS*........  brown rice, millet, whole
                 wheat and/or rye berries,
                 barley, corn meal, rolled
                 oats, rye flakes, bulghur
                 (cracked wheat), buckwheat
MISCELLANEOUS*.  sugar-free jams, mayo-
                 naise, ketchup (sometimes
                 called "table sauce"),
                 popcorn, miso, agar agar
                 kuzu. (Refrigerate all ex-
                 cept kuzu and agar agar.)
NOODLES*.......  whole wheat, buckwheat,
                 Jerusalem artichoke.
NUTRITIONAL....  nutritional yeast, bran,
SUPPLEMENTS*     vacuum packed wheat germ,
                 rice polishings, etc.
NUTS & SEEDS*..  almonds, sunflower, chia,
                 flax, sesame, pumpkin,
                 alfalfa (to sprout), etc.
OILS*..........  cold pressed olive, sun-
                 flower, sesame, walnut,
                 soy.
SOUPS..........  vegetable powders and
                 bouillon cubes.
SWEETENERS.....  honey, maple syrup,
                 molasses, barley malt,
                 rice bran syrup
                 unsweetened carob powder.
SEAWEED........  dulse, wakame, nori, etc.
```

* Refrigerate. See "Natural Food Kitchen
Hints", pp.299-301.

STAPLES, CONT.

## GROUP B - PURCHASE ONCE A WEEK

BREAD*......... whole grain home-made, or
               good store-bought.
BUTTER*........ unsalted dairy butter and
               seed butters, such as
               tahini or almond butter.
EGGS*.......... organic.
FREEZER ITEMS*. chicken, fish, nut/seed
               burgers.
VEGETABLES*.... Those that keep well:
               potatoes, carrots, radish,
               parsnips, turnips, sun-
               chokes (Jerusalem arti-
               chokes), squash.
FRUITS*........ Those that keep well:
               apples, pears and other
               hard fruits.

* Refrigerate. See "Natural Food Kitchen
Hints", pp.299-301.

As you can see, this is quite an
extensive list, even though it does not
include the third category of staples - the
more perishable foods (leafy greens and the
more delicate fruits and vegetables)! With
such a variety of foods from this staples
list, - whole grains, noodles, beans, nuts
and seeds, frozen chicken and fish, certain
vegetables and fruits, and condiments and
flavorings, - many different delicious meals
can be created with very little daily
shopping. This saves time and food waste, and
stimulates your own creative instincts.

CHAPTER 7

PLANNING YOUR MEALS

In planning your meals there are a few basic considerations to keep in mind:

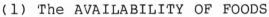

(1) The AVAILABILITY OF FOODS
(2) The COST OF FOOD
(3) SPOILAGE
(4) PREPARATION TIME
(5) FOR WHOM ARE YOU COOKING?
(6) THE CLIMATE
(7) CALORIES
(8) The OVER-ALL PLAN of the meal, which should include good taste, moderation, simplicity, balance, variety and vitality.
(9) The BASIC FOOD ELEMENTS included in a daily menu - protein, vitamins, minerals, oils, fiber, chlorophyll.
(10) PROPORTIONS OF FOOD CATEGORIES: How many vegetables, fruits, proteins to include in a day.
(11) COMBINING VEGETARIAN PROTEINS to increase net protein utilization. See Chapter 8.
(12) How to COMBINE AND CONSUME FOODS for better digestion and assimilation. See Chapter 9.

Planning your foods well simply means using your common sense. Learn to develop your ability to listen to the magical voice inside you.

In planning your meals, it is important to consider the availability of the foods, the cost and spoilage factors, preparation time, and "cooking for others". These issues are discussed in Section 1, Common Conflicts.

In addition, the following factors should be considered:

## CLIMATE

Your body will adapt more easily to a new diet if you choose "lighter" foods (such as more fruits and vegetables) in summer, and "heavier" foods (such as whole grains and beans) in winter. If possible, use foods that are grown in your region. Those foods have within them all that is needed to survive in that climate, and that factor is transferred to you.

## CALORIES

Foods are likely to be high in calories if they are:

(1) Greasy or oily: Butter; fried foods, such as potato chips or french fries; foods that are cooked in large amounts of fat.

(2) Smooth and thick: Rich sauces, cream cheese, sour cream, nut butters (tahini, almond butter), cream.

(3) Sweet and gooey: candy, regular soft drinks, rich baked goods, ice cream.

(4) Alcoholic.

A food is less likely to be high in calories if it is:
(1) Thin and watery, like tomato juice.
(2) Crisp (but not greasy crisp), like celery, radish, cucumber, melon, and many other fresh, raw fruits and vegetables.
(3) Bulky, like salad greens.

When considering the caloric value of foods, it is also important to consider how they affect the metabolism.
"Junk" foods, particularly foods made from processed flour and sugar, are the worst offenders for putting on weight. They are high in calories, and often contain large amounts of "hidden" salt and sugar (See Appendix -Hidden Sugars and Hidden Salt, pp.306 and 307.).
In addition to being high in calories, "junk" foods are low in nutrients, and replace more nutritious foods which would help balance the metabolism.
Certain "Foods to Enjoy", such as nuts and seeds and nut butters and whole grains, are high in calories, but also provide essential nutrients important for balancing the body. They also provide fiber, which aids in elimination and therefore over-all health. Quality fats, such as nuts and seeds and certain oils, also provide a gradual release of energy, which helps cut down on cravings.

As you cut out "junk" food and your metabolism begins to balance out, your weight may begin to stabilize. Your body should become stronger and slimmer naturally.

A MEAL PLAN

When we are first making a conscious effort to have a diet plan, it helps to be aware of how we have been eating up to now. To assist you in becoming aware of your eating habits, fill out a chart for a week, with a format something like the one below:

| DAILY DIET REPORT | | | | | | | |
|---|---|---|---|---|---|---|---|
| | 1st Day | 2nd Day | 3rd Day | 4th Day | 5th Day | 6th day | 7th Day |
| Morning Meal | | | | | | | |
| Noon Meal | | | | | | | |
| Evening Meal | | | | | | | |
| Snacks | | | | | | | |
| Comments | | | | | | | |

Filling out the "Comments" can help expand your awareness of the effects of your diet on your over-all health. This column can include reactions you may have after a meal - physical symptoms, including sleepiness, or emotional swings. You may want to note circumstances surrounding the meal, including eating under stress, fighting at a meal, etc. Working with this column can help you discover food allergies, and help you better understand food cravings and your relationship with your food.

When you plan your meal, key points to keep in mind are Good Taste, Moderation Balance, Simplicity, Variety and Vitality.

## Good Taste

Don't just eat food because it's healthy. Make it delicious, and appetizing.

## Moderation

When giving up meat, milk, salt and sugar, don't "overdo" on nuts, cheese, tofu (soy bean curd. See "Glossary"), soy sauce, honey, molasses, yogurt and whole wheat bread. Be moderate. Overconsumption of these foods (i.e., every day or twice a day), can encourage mucous build up, digestive stress, allergies or other stress reactions.

## Balance

Balance your meals by using their color, texture, flavor and shape. This is Mother Nature's way of helping you get a good range and balance of food value, as well as making it more appealing to the eye and taste buds.

## Simplicity

Use the "KISS" Rule: Keep It Simple, Sweetheart.
Preparing 2-3 items per meal will be easiest on your digestion, time and energy.
Although it is always best to prepare foods fresh, sometimes making extra for the next day will cut down on stress, and help prevent one from eating "junk" food. See Section 1, "Preparation Time", p.17.

## Variety

Most deficiency diseases result from not getting enough variety in the diet, rather than a lack of one specific nutrient.

Vary your vegetables, fruits, grains, nuts and seeds and oils from day to day. (See "Foods to Enjoy" for lists of the varieties to include. Also see the "Appendix" for meal plan ideas.) This makes your meals more interesting, gives you a greater balance of nutrients, and helps prevent food allergies (sometimes aggrevated from eating a food too much and too often - see "Foods to Avoid", "Allergens", p.55.)

Sometimes we are not aware of how often we repeat the same foods over and over. (Filling out the diet plan for one week helps this awareness.) This is usually because we don't have the time or energy to experiment with something different.

Learning a few basic techniques, such as those outlined in Chapter 10, can free you from the stress of thinking about recipes, yet leave room for variety.

## Vitality

Choose foods that give you vitality - the "Foods to Enjoy" listed in Chapter 1, and in Columns (2) and (3) of the "Transition Chart" (page 59).

FOOD ELEMENTS FOR A DAILY MENU

In planning your meal, be sure it pro-provides you with the following elements:

| Element | Food Source |
|---------|-------------|
| enzymes | raw food, sprouts. |
| fiber | whole grains, bran, raw fruits and vegetables, sprouts. |
| chlorophyll | raw greens, alfalfa sprouts. |
| protein | lamb, chicken, fish, eggs, cheese, yogurt, beans, whole grains, sprouts, nuts and seeds, mixed raw vegetables. |
| vitamins | all of the above, and lightly steamed vegetables |
| minerals | all of the above, and lightly steamed vegetables |
| quality oils | nuts and seeds, avocados, cold pressed oils (see list under Foods to Enjoy) |

PROPORTIONS OF FOOD CATEGORIES IN A DAY

To support over-all good health, include in a day's meal the following proportions of food types:

4 to 5 Vegetables in a day
At first glance, this may seem like a lot of vegetables, but consider that in a salad alone you can easily have many varieties. Make a "rainbow salad".

Include a good portion of your vegetables in a raw state, since this is where you will get most of your enzymes and fiber. If possible, 60% raw foods is good.

### 1 to 2 Fruits in a Day
Enjoy any fruits in great variety, limiting only the citrus. Citrus can be overly-acid and overly-cleansing, although the freshly picked are less acidic.

### 1 to 2 Proteins in a Day
The type and amount of protein, as with the diet in general, depends upon each individual - their over-all health status (including any special situation such as pregnancy), age, body size, climate, type and amount of activity and stress.

The amount of protein per day varies from 25 to 70 grams, depending on the individual and the type of food, the usable protein available and its digestibility.

The primary types of protein are meat, including fish and chicken, dairy, eggs, nuts and seeds, sprouts, whole grains, beans and peas.

In choosing which types of protein are best for you, it is wise to take into consideration your over-all health status and the state of your digestion. You may need the more concentrated "flesh" protein, or you may find you are not able to fully digest meat. When proteins are not digested and assimilated properly, they rot, become toxic and put tremendous stress on the body.

If you have decided to cut down on meat consumption, begin by switching to fish and chicken, and eating less meat in general. Most Americans eat more meat than they can use, and this causes stress on their digestion and elimination.

---

1-2 proteins per day can include any of the types of protein which are best suited to your taste and nutritional needs. In general, however, meat protein would not be recommended twice a day. If you are depending solely on vegetarian proteins, two per day would probably be advisable. (For example, bean sprouts and nuts and seeds included in one meal, and grains and beans at another meal.)

Consult with your nutrition consultant or physician concerning your protein needs.

CHAPTER 8

PROTEIN IN A VEGETARIAN DIET

Nuts and seeds, sprouts, whole grains, beans and peas can provide adequate protein, especially when eaten in certain combinations within a period of 12-16 hours. (See Protein Combining, which follows). They are also more economical than meat, are high in fiber and low in fat, and are less likely to contain toxic additives.

Don't depend on cheese and tofu for your protein. Over-abundance of these types of protein can be congesting. Vary your proteins, and learn how to combine them.

Nuts and seeds, beans and grains can be sprouted or eaten in certain combinations to increase the protein utilized from these foods.

Sprouting increases the nutrient value of a nut, seed, legume or grain and also pre-digests the protein so that it is more fully assimilated.

Combining nuts and seeds, beans and peas, whole grains and dairy at the same meal,[1] or at least within 12-16 hours, can also increase the amount of utilizable protein assimilated from each of the foods.

A simple formula to use is called "Slugem". This formula is a way to remember the letters S-L-G-M, the first letters of the words Seeds, Legumes (beans), Grains and Milk products. Combining foods in the following orders of sequence will give you a more complete protein:

Combining Seeds or nuts with Legumes makes a more complete protein.
Combining Legumes with Grains makes a more complete protein.
Combining Grains with Milk products makes a more complete protein.

Combining seeds and/or nuts with grains increases the net protein utilized, but is not quite as complete as the other combinations.

On the next page is a list of foods to help you in combining. Note that each category also includes the by-products made from the particular kind of food. For example, included with seeds are seed/nut butters and seed/nut milks.

```
☆☆☆☆☆☆☆☆ COMBINING PROTEINS ☆☆☆☆☆☆☆☆
SEEDS & NUTS  +  LEGUMES (BEANS)  +  GRAINS  +  MILK

sesame seeds     lentils              rice          milk
tahini (sesame   split peas           millet        cheese
  butter)        soy beans            barley        yogurt
almonds          mung beans           oats          kefir
almond butter    other beans and      buckwheat
sunflower seeds    peas               rye
pumpkin seeds    bean flour, such     other grains
flax seeds         as soy flour       grain flour
walnuts          soy products:        noodles
pecans             soy sauce          grain milk
other nuts         miso               whole grain
  and seeds        tofu                 bread &
nut milks          tempeh             crackers
                     ☆☆☆☆☆☆☆☆☆☆
```

READING THIS CHART:
   Eaten within 16 hours, the following combinations
of foods will together make a complete protein:

   Seeds & Nuts + Legumes      = complete protein
   Legumes       + Grains      = complete protein
   Grains        + Milk products = complete protein

   Nuts and Seeds plus grains is a more complete protein than either nuts and seeds alone, or grains alone,
but is not as complete a protein as the combinations on
this chart.
   To remember the combinations, think of the key
phrase "slug-em" (the power-punch of protein), standing
for the letters "S" (seeds) + "L" (legumes) + "G"
(grains) + "M" (milk products).

## NOTES & EXAMPLES:

   (1) In general, combine 3 parts grain to 1
part legume.
(2) Adding a small amount of bean flour to
grain flour increases the protein used. Even
as little as 2 Tablespoons of soy flour added
to 3 cups of whole wheat or rye flour in-
increases the net protein utilized.

   (3) Examples of good combinations are:
     (a) Miso/Tahini spread on a rice cracker
     (b) Tofu + noodles with tahini sauce

     At the same meal:
     (c) Split pea soup and "sunburgers"
     (d) Lentil soup and a rice casserole
     (e) Glass of nut milk and a tofu dip on
         mixed raw vegetables.

CHAPTER 9


## COMBINING AND CONSUMING FOODS FOR BETTER DIGESTION

Ideally, we should be able to eat foods in any combination at any time of the day, and digest them well. Many people, however, experience digestive stress in the forms of gas, bloating, poor or infrequent bowel movements, over all fatigue, etc. For them, it is of first importance to find out why the digestive capacity is weak. Consult with your nutrition consultant or doctor.

Until your digestion is strong again, it is often helpful to avoid eating certain types and combinations of foods which don't digest as easily, and even to be aware of how and when to eat.


## TYPES OF FOODS

When first changing your diet, raw foods can sometimes be irritating, and you may experience gas. You can blend the foods, grate them, or lightly steam a portion of them, especially the "harder" vegetables. (Try to have some leafy greens raw, each day, however.)

Other types of foods can in and of themselves be "gassy", such as cabbage, broccoli, garlic, onions, brussel sprouts, peppers, and beans. Beans can be blended, or cooked in a special way to cut down on the "gassy" effect. See Recipes - Beans.

Nuts and seeds and dried fruit also need to be broken down well, by soaking or blending, and by chewing well.

FOOD COMBINING FOR EASIER DIGESTION

You may already have seen several charts on food combining, all different. However, I find that certain basic combinations eaten at the same meal can cause stress. They are the following:

OFTEN DIFFICULT COMBINATIONS:

(1) Certain Protein Foods + Starch:

> Meat + Starch (except fish + rice)
> > for example, meat plus potatoes, grain or bread
>
> Nuts and seeds, and nut butters + starch (except ground nuts and seeds and nut milks)
> > for example, nut butter on bread
>
> Eggs + Starch
> > for example, eggs + bread, or eggs + cereal
>
> Cheese + Starch
> > for example, cheese on bread, or cheese + noodles

(2) Certain Protein Foods + Fruit (except tomatoes and the tropical fruits, such as papaya, mango and pineapple):

> Meat + Fruit (except tomatoes)
> Nuts & Seeds + Fruit
> Eggs + Fruit
> Dairy + Fruit
> > for example, yogurt + fruit, or cheese + fruit

Some people also have difficulty combining fruits with vegetables (except tomatoes, avocados and the tropical fruits).

EASILY DIGESTED COMBINATIONS:

In general, the best combinations for those with delicate digestion are the following:

    Meat + Vegetables
    Starch + Vegetables
    Fruit is best eaten by itself
    Melons are best eaten alone

Sometimes soaked raisins and fresh bananas combine well with starch such as cereals and breads.

Tomatoes and avocados, although fruits, combine well with vegetables and meats.

How long do you wait before you can eat another category of food that does not combine well? It depends on the individual, but basically when you feel hungry again. Usually, you need to wait at least 1/2 hour after eating fruit before another type of food, and 1 to 1 1/2 hours after protein before eating starch or fruit.

Try to space your dessert sometime after your main course if they are poor combinations.

Please note that it is most important to find out why the digestive capacity is weak. Avoiding difficult combinations of foods helps give the body a rest, but is not a solution.

## TIMING OF FOODS FOR BETTER DIGESTION AND ASSIMILATION

Most people feel better when they eat a power-packed breakfast, a light dinner and an in-between lunch. (Breakfast like a king, lunch like a prince, and dinner like a pauper).

It is not necessary to have a large breakfast. However, to sustain your energy throughout the day, it helps to have a breakfast that is high in protein, and low in sweets. Sometimes even grains, such as oatmeal, for breakfast can be too sweet for some people, leaving them fatigued mid-morning or afternoon. (This could be an "allergic" reaction.) Topping your cereals with nut milk, and having a green salad with the cereal may help combat this reaction.

Those with delicate digestion, or blood sugar imbalance, often find that they cannot digest more concentrated proteins, such as beans and meats, as well after 3:00 in the afternoon. For them, having that type of protein earlier in the day helps combat digestive stress and fatigue.

See "Appendix", p.309, for "Planned Menu" ideas.

## EATING TO AID DIGESTION

Eating your food without stress can be the most important factor in digesting and assimilating all the nutrients possible. Be aware of the following:

(1) Eat only when you are hungry.

(2) Do not feel you must eat when you are sick. It is generally best Not to eat, especially if you do not feel like it!

(3) It is best not to eat when you are tired or have negative emotions such as anger, guilt, fear, etc. Negativity makes your body tense, and inhibits all proper functioning. If you are under stress all the time, try to let it go during meals. This is a special time to nourish yourself on many levels.

(4) When you are ready to eat, take a few moments, center yourself, put all your cares aside, and allow yourself this time to relax and enjoy your meal.

(5) Consume foods and water as close to room temperature as possible. Extremes of hot or cold are a shock to the system, and can inhibit the production of digestive enzymes.

(6) Try not to slouch or wear tight clothing while you eat, as this can inhibit proper digestion.

(7) Don't wash your food down with water. Many people find they digest better if they do not take any liquids with meals. If you are thirsty while you eat, chew and swallow your food first, then sip your water.

(8) CHEW extremely well! It is in the chewing process that digestion begins. Chewing not only breaks food down, but stimulates the production of digestive enzymes.

(9) DON'T OVER-EAT! Eat until you're satisfied, but not stuffed. This is essential for good health.

CHAPTER 10

BASIC FOOD PREPARATION

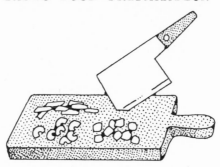

An unexpected bonus which many people experience when they switch to vital foods is the joy in the preparation itself. It is a touch with Nature that is especially rare in city life, a way of making contact with the earth and its nourishing life force.

As you are becoming accustomed to new, healthier forms of food preparation, it may at first seem more complicated and time consuming than the methods you have been using. Be patient. This is a learning experience, and it always takes time at first to learn new ways of food preparation. Soon you will be amazed at how much simpler and more delicious healthy eating is.

Remember that in preparing quality meals, you are choosing increased health and vitality for you and your family.

A good health-maintenance program includes stress-free food preparation. This means (1) fast and easy preparation; and, (2) preserving the nutrients in your foods during the preparation.

FAST AND EASY FOOD PREPARATION

There are many ways to cut down on the time and energy it takes to prepare meals. (Also see "Section 1, Common Conflicts - Preparation Time", pp.17-20):

* Arrange your kitchen well.
* Purchase time-saving equipment and utensils (See pp.68-71).
* Keep in mind an over-all food plan (See pp.77-85).
* Have basic staples on hand ( See pp.74-76.). Include foods that cook quickly, such as rolled oats, whole grain noodles, kasha, fish, eggs, etc. Also have on hand staples that add flavor or texture to last minute cooking, such as garlic, onions, ginger, miso, tahini, kuzu, soup bouillons, etc. Also include some root vegetables, which may take longer to cook, but keep well and may save you a trip to the vegetable market.
* Keep some pre-prepared foods in the refrigerator or freezer to be ready to use in a variety of ways. For example, have on hand spreads, dips or dressings, sprouts, "sunburgers", lentil walnut burgers, cooked brown rice, cooked beans, cooked chicken, sauerkraut, washed and cut leafy greens and vegetables (although this is generally not advised, since washing and cutting results in a loss of nutrients).
* Use recipes that are easy and quick. The recipes in this book are very easy, but some are faster than others. Refer to the lists "Quick Foods", pp.338-339, and "Snacks to Go for Work or Travel", p.337, in the Special Index.
* Learn fast-cooking techniques, such as those which follow. (Note that these techniques are described more fully in each recipe section.)

## FAST-COOKING TECHNIQUES

Most people find that using specific recipes requires more planning and shopping ahead, organization and time than they can afford.

It is simpler to refer to recipes for ideas, and then create a meal with ingredients that are on hand, easy to find, and that fit one's particular tastes and nutritional requirements. Learning a few fast-cooking techniques such as the following gives you this freedom. The skeletan of a technique allows for more variety and creativity without excessive shopping and planning ahead.

### Nut Milks
Blend ground nuts and seeds, or nut/seed butter, such as tahini or almond butter, with water. Add pure sweeteners, flavorings or "Bulk" ingredients. (See "Nut Milks", pp.154-156.)

### Basic Soup
Add to a broth any of the following in any combinations: lightly steamed vegetables, cooked chicken or fish, cooked grains,noodles or beans, chopped parsley, chopped tomatoes. (See "Soups", p.171.)

### Blended Soups
Raw or lightly cooked vegetables, or cooked beans or grains can be blended with hot or cold water or juice, plus spices, to make wonderful soups. (See p.185.)

### Blended Cereals
Left over grains, such as rice, millet or barley, can be blended with hot water or nut milk and seasonings for a quick, hearty breakfast. (See p.134.)

## Blended Sauces

Cooked grains or beans can be blended with hot water and spices, miso or tahini for a quick sauce. (See p.208.)

## Blended Dressings

Raw vegetables can be blended with olive oil, lemon juice or apple cider vinegar and spices for a quick dressing. (See p.201.)

## Grain Pilaf

Grains, nuts and seeds and lentils or split peas can be cooked in any combinations in a broth, adding vegetables in the last couple of minutes of cooking. (See p.254.)

## Meal in One Sauté

Lightly sauté on a low heat in olive oil or butter with any spices, any of the following in any combinations: cooked grain, beans or noodles, lightly steamed or raw vegetables, cooked chicken or fish. Add ground nuts and seeds and a quick sauce.

## Quick Steam Soup or Meal In a Pot

Soups or whole meals can be created by steaming ingredients over a broth. (Other foods, such as noodles or fish, can meanwhile be cooking in the broth under the steamer.) For a soup, add the steamed ingredients to the broth. For a meal, separate the ingredients from the broth. For delicious examples, refer to Create-A-Soup, p.178, and Create-A-Meal, p.226.

## Simple Salad

Mix raw or lightly steamed vegetables with cooked chicken, cooked beans , cooked noodles or cooked grains. Top with a dressing.

## PREPARING FOODS TO PRESERVE NUTRIENTS

Foods should be prepared as close to eating time as possible. The longer you wait to eat foods after they have been washed, sliced and cooked, the more nutrients will have been lost.[1]

To preserve nutrients and fiber in foods, prepare foods with as little heat as is reasonable for that particular food. Enzyme destruction begins at 130°. Also, with high heat cooking, proteins become more difficult to digest or less available to the body, many vitamins and minerals are lost and fiber becomes less well utilizable.[2]

Never fry foods on high heats, since oils can become toxic at high heats, and fried, barbequed fats are carcinogenic (cancer causing).[3] Use low heats when "sautée-ing". Use olive oil or butter for cooking, since it takes a higher heat for those oils to become toxic than for other oils.

Digestibility of fats is reduced when they are cooked beyond 250°.[4]

See each individual recipe section for low heat cooking techniques, and see "Kitchen Hints" for a few other tips.


You will note that not all the recipes in this book adhere strictly to low heat cooking. This takes into consideration "transition cooking". That is, someone, who has never before cooked brown rice will probably be more at ease cooking it the fast higher heat way (although the low heat cooking technique is also given). Many other recipes, although perhaps not as full of vitality as the low heat or raw food recipes presented in this book, are delicious introductions to healthful eating.

# SECTION III

******** R E C I P E S ********

THE BEST RECIPE

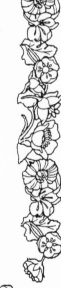

| | |
|---|---|
| 4 handfuls Friendship | 1 pound Courage |
| 3 cups Loyalty | 3 ounces Tenderness |
| 4 cups Honesty | 3 cups Forgiveness |
| 6 ounces Compassion | 1 gallon Gratitude |
| 2 quarts Peace | 1 bushel Faith |
| 1 gallon Love | 1 barrel Laughter |

Adjust measurements to your own needs.

Gently mix Friendship, Loyalty & Honesty.
Blend in Compassion.
Fold in Peace.
Sweeten with Love.
Spice with Courage.
Kneed with Tenderness.
Let rise with Forgiveness & Gratitude.
Bind together with Faith.
Lace with a Song.
Sprinkle abundantly with Laughter.

Warm in the sunshine.

Slice with a prayer.
Share with a friend, and devour.

Serve daily with generous helpings.
Serves multitudes.
Keeps forever, and gets better with age.

******** NOTES FOR RECIPES ********

In reading recipes, please note the following guidelines:

* Use the purest of foods whenever possible:

    Oils: raw, cold pressed. For olive, use raw green or a light virgin olive oil
    Eggs: organic
    Chicken: organically raised, free-range
    Butter: unsalted; raw, if possible
    Honey: raw, unfiltered, organic
    Molasses: unsulphured
    Maple syrup: pure, unpasteurized
    Carob powder: raw, unsweetened
    Dried fruit: unsulphured, untreated
    Soy sauce: Use those with no toxic additives, such as MSG. Use wheat-free, if allergic to wheat. The wheat-free soy sauce often has a stronger taste, so you may need to use less than indicated.
    Apple Cider Vinegar: unpasteurized, organically made
    Water: spring, or, if recommended by a nutrition consultant or doctor, use distilled
    Vanilla extract: pure
    Baking powder: aluminum free
    Tofu: made without toxic additives.

* Cook with olive oil or butter. For salads use cold pressed olive, sesame, sunflower, avocado, almond, flax, walnut or soy. "Sauté" means lightly stirring on a low heat.

* When using cayenne pepper, add it after cooking. High heats kill some of the valuable nutrients. When used raw, it is said to have strengthening properties. It is hot tasting, so add it gradually.

## ABBREVIATIONS OF MEASUREMENTS

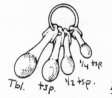

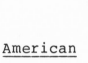 American

| | | | | | |
|---|---|---|---|---|---|
| tsp. | = | teaspoon(s) | pt. | = | pint(s) |
| Tbl. | = | Tablespoon(s) | qt. | = | quart(s) |
| c. | = | cup(s) | gal. | = | gallon(s) |
| oz. | = | ounce(s) | lb. | = | pound(s) |

### Metric

| | | |
|---|---|---|
| g. | = | gram(s) |
| L. | = | Liter(s) |
| mL. | = | milliliter(s) |

## AMERICAN AND METRIC EQUIVALENTS

AMERICAN                    METRIC

**Liquid Volume Equivalents**

| | |
|---|---|
| 1/5 tsp. | 1 milliliter |
| 1 tsp. | 5 milliliters |
| 1 fluid ounce | 30 milliliters |
| 1 cup (8 oz.) | 250 milliliters |
| 1 pint (2 cups) | 500 milliliters |
| 1 quart (2 pints) | 1 liter |
| 1 gallon (4 qts.) | 4 liters |

**Weight Equivalents**

| | |
|---|---|
| 1 ounce | 30 grams, or 16 drams |
| 1 pound (16 ozs.) | 454 grams |
| 2 pounds | 1 kilogram |

********** LIQUID VOLUME EQUIVALENTS **********

| tsp. | Tbl. | Fluid oz. | cup | pints | quarts | gallons | metric |
|---|---|---|---|---|---|---|---|
| 1/5 tsp. = | | | | | | | = 1 ML |
| 1 tsp. = | 1/3 Tbl. | = 60 drops | | | | | = 5 ML |
| 3 tsp. = | 1 Tbl. | | | | | | = 15 ML |
| 6 tsp. = | 2 Tbl. | = 1 oz. | | | | | = 30 ML |
| 12 tsp. = | 4 Tbl. | = 2 oz. | = 1/4 c. | | | | |
| 16 tsp. = | 5 1/3 Tbl. or 5 Tbl.+ 1 tsp. | = 2 2/3 oz. | = 1/3 c. | | | | |
| 18 tsp. = | 6 Tbl. | = 3 oz. | = 3/8 c. or 1/4 c.+ 2 Tbl. | | | | |
| 24 tsp. = | 8 Tbl. | = 4 oz. | = 1/2 c. | | | | |
| 26 tsp. = | 10 Tbl. | = 5 oz. | = 5/8 c. or 1/2 c.+ 2 Tbl. | | | | |
| 36 tsp. = | 12 Tbl. | = 6 oz. | = 3/4 c. | | | | |
| 42 tsp. = | 14 Tbl. | = 7 oz. | = 7/8 c. or 3/4 c.+ 2 Tbl. | | | | |
| 48 tsp. = | 16 Tbl. | = 8 oz. | = 1 c. | = 1/2 pt. | | | = 240 ML |
| 96 tsp. = | 32 Tbl. | = 16 oz. | = 2 c. | = 1 pt. | | | = 480 ML |
| 192 tsp. = | 64 Tbl. | = 32 oz. | = 4 c. | = 2 pt. | = 1 qt. | | = 1 liter |
| 768 tsp. = | 256 Tbl. | = 128 oz. | = 16 c. | = 4 pt. | = 4 qt. | = 1 gal. | = 4 liter |

COMMON FOOD EQUIVALENTS

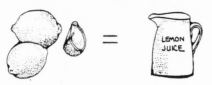

```
Almonds, unblanched, whole......1 c.  .....= 6 oz.
         unblanched, ground.....2 2/3 c. ..= 1 lb.
         unblanched, slivered...5 2/3 c. ..= 1 lb.
         blanched, whole........1 c.  .....= 5 1/3 oz.
         unblanched, whole .....20 nuts ...= 1 oz.
                                           = 4 Tbl. meal
Apple, fresh, peeled, chopped ..5-6 c. ....= 2 lbs. whole
         dried, chopped, packed,1 c. ......= 4 1/2 oz.
Apricots, dried ................3 c. ......= 1 lb.
         cooked, drained .......3 c. ......= 1 lb.
Bananas, 3-4 medium sized, whole...........= 1 lb.
         mashed.............................= 2 c.
Barley ..................... 3 c. ......= 1 lb.
                            1 c. ......= 4 c. cooked
Beans, uncooked, in general ....2 1/2 c....= 1 lb.
         chick peas.............3 c. ......= 1 lb.
         kidney beans ..........1 1/2 c. ..= 1 lb.
                                           = 9 c. cooked
         lentils ...............3 c. ......= 1 lb.
         lima beans ............2 1/3 c. ..= 1 lb.
                                           = 6 c. cooked
         navy beans ............2 1/3 c. ..= 1 lb.
         split peas ............3 c. ......= 1 lb.
Bean sprouts ...................3/4 c. ....= 15 oz.
Blueberries, whole ...........2 c. ......= 3/4 lb.
Bran ...........................4 c. ......= 1/2 lb.
Brown Rice ...................2 1/2 c. ..= 1 lb.
                            1/3 c. ....= 1 c. cooked
Buckwheat ......................1 c. ......= 3 c. cooked
Bulgar .........................4 c. ......= 1 1/3 lb.
Butter .........................1 stick ...= 8 Tbl.
                                           = 1/2 c.
                            4 sticks ..= 2 c.
                                           = 1 lb.
Carrot, 2 large, sliced ........2 1/2 c. ..= 14 oz.
         grated ................10 c. .....= 2 lbs.
Celery, 2 medium sized or 1 large stalk ...= 1 c. chopped
Cheese, fresh grated ...........5 c. ......= 1 lb.
Cottage Cheese .................1 c. ......= 1/2 lb.
Coconut, fine grated ...........3 1/2 oz.  = 1 c.
         shredded ..............5 c. ......= 1 lb.
Cornmeal .......................3 c. ......= 1 lb.
                            1 c. ......= 4 c. cooked
Currants .......................5 c. ......= 1 1/2 lb.
```

Common Food Equivalents, cont.

```
Dates, pitted ..................2 1/2 c. ..= 1 lb.
                               18 dates ..= 1/3 c.
Eggs, hen, large, whole ........5 .........= 1 c., about
           medium .............6 .........= 1 c., about
           small ..............7 .........= 1 c., about
           egg whites .........8 - 10 ....= 12 c.
           egg yolks ..........12 - 14 ...= 1 c.
Flour .........................4 c. ......= 1 lb.
Herbs, dried ..................1/3-1/2 tsp= 1 Tbl. fresh
Honey .........................1 1/2 c. ..= 1 lb.
Lemon .........................1 .........= 2-3 Tbl. juice
                                         = 2 tsp. rind
                               1 tsp.juice= 1/2 tsp.vinegar
Lime ..........................1 .........= 1 1/2 to 2 Tbl.
                                                  juice
Molasses ......................1 c. ......= 13 oz.
Mushrooms, sliced .............4 c. ......= 10 oz.
Noodles, uncooked .............1 c. ......= 1 3/4 c. cooked
Nuts, in the shell:
           almonds, walnuts ...1 1/2 c. ..= 1 lb.
           peanuts, pecans ....2 1/4 c. ..= 1 lb.
Nuts, shelled .................1 c. ......= 1 c. ground
           pecans .............2 c. ......= 7 1/2 oz.
                               6 c. ......= 1 1/2 lb.
Oats, rolled ..................4 3/4 c. ..= 1 lb.
Onion, 1 medium sized, peeled, chopped.....= 1 c.
Orange ........................1 medium ..= 7 Tbl. juice
                                         = 2 1/2 Tbl. rind
Pepper, fresh green or red bell, chopped...= 1 1/4 c.
Pineapple, fresh, skinned, chopped, 2 c. ..= 1 lb.
Potatoes, raw, unpeeled ........1 lb. .....= 2 c. mashed
                                         = 3 c. chopped
Powdered Milk .................3 c. ......= 1/2 lb.
Prunes, pitted ................2 1/2 c. ..= 1 lb.
           cooked, drained ....2 c. ......= 1 lb.
Raisins, seeded, whole ........3 1/4 c. ..= 1 lb.
Scallion, 2 medium sized, chopped .........= 1/4 c.
Sesame Seeds, hulled ..........4 c. ......= 1 lb.
Sunflower Seeds, hulled .......4 c. ......= 1 lb.
Tofu ..........................2 c. ......= 1 lb.
Tomatoes, 2 large chopped .................= 3-4 c.
Water .........................2 c. ......= 1 lb.
Wheat Germ ....................2 1/4 c. ..= 1/2 lb.
Winter squash, 1 large, cooked ............= 4 c.
Yeast, dry ....................4 Tbl. ....= 1 oz.
Yogurt ........................2 1/4 c. ..= 1 lb.
Zucchini, 1 large sliced ..................= 1 1/2 c.
```

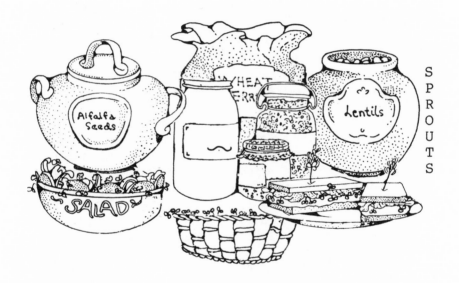

******** S P R O U T S ********

Sprouts are, very simply, a sprouted seed, bean or grain. They are the most vital and nourishing of all foods.

Sprouts are high in essential nutrients, are a good source of dietary fiber, low in calories, inexpensive and easy to prepare. Depending on the sprout, they contain varying amounts of Vitamins A, B Complex, C, D, E and K, factors G and U, and minerals such as calcium, magnesium, phosphorus, chlorine, potassium, iron, zinc and silicon.

Many sprouts contain all 8 essential amino acids, which means that they are a good source of protein. The net protein utilized can be increased by combining certain sprouts, such as mung and lentil, at the same meal.

Sprouting increases the nutrient value of a seed. Vitamins C, B and E increase 10% to 30%, and the amount of protein can increase up to 1200%.[1]

Sprouting also predigests the protein, making it more easily digested and assimilated, and breaks down the starch molecules into simple sugars, making sprouts a good energy food.

-108-

SECTION III, RECIPES, "SPROUTS"

---

Sprouts can be added to any dish, such as sandwiches, salads, omelettes, cereals, breads, blender drinks, sauces, etc. Try not to cook them, as heat will destroy many of its valuable nutrients and vitality.


HOW TO SPROUT

A seed holds within it the blueprint of life - all necessary elements for normal health and growth. Add to it water, air and sunshine, and a sprout will burst forth.

Sprouts are available in any health food store and in many supermarkets. They are also fun to grow at home. It's easy to do, very inexpensive, and a great thrill to watch the little seeds grow into beautiful, delicious salad greens.

(Children enjoy growing sprouts, and love to eat them, too. This is a great way to introduce them to the miracle of growing things, to have fun doing it, and to eat something super-packed with nutrition.)

A variety of different types of seeds, beans or grains can be sprouted. See "Sprouting Chart". If you have never sprouted before, try alfalfa for an easy beginning. Use seeds which have not been sprayed with chemicals. Purchase them at the health food store.

Three good ways to sprout will be described in the pages that follow:

(1) The traditional "jar" method, useful for sprouting seeds, beans or grains;

(2) The "basket" method, devised by Steve Meyerowitz ("Sproutman"). This method is best suited to sprouting seeds, such as alfalfa, fenugreek, clover and radish. It is not as suitable for sprouting grains or beans.

(3) The "bag" method, also devised by Sproutman, is great for sprouting grains and beans, but is not as suitable for seeds.

With the "jar" method, the seed, bean or grain is soaked and sprouted in the jar. With the "basket" method, the soaked seeds are transferred to a basket where they "root" themselves to the weave of the basket and grow straight toward the light. With the "bag" method, grains or beans are soaked and grown in a flaxseed bag.

When you begin sprouting, you will be amazed at how few seeds you need to produce a quantity of sprouts. They expand at least 8 times their present size, so be sure the jar or bag is large enough to accomodate the increase, and that you do not use too many seeds.
For alfalfa seeds, 2 Tablespoons for a quart size jar is good. If you use the basket method, use 3 Tablespoons for a 6" basket, 4 Tablespoons for a 8" basket or 5 Tablespoons for a 9" basket. One to ten cups of grains or beans can be sprouted in the flaxseed bag, depending on the size of the bag.

When you soak the seeds, use spring water, as the seeds will absorb the water. It is not as important to use spring water for rinsing. Never use hot water, as it will sterilize the seeds and cause them to rot.

The time it takes for a sprout to reach maturity depends on the type of seed, the temperature of the weather, and the humidity. When it is hot, rinse more frequently, to cool the seeds and to prevent mold.
Sprouts are generally ready when they are between 1/4 and 1 1/2" long. The sprout is past its peak when the second leaf system begins. Alfalfa sprouts are best at 1" long, and grain sprouts are ready when the length of the sprout equals the length of the grain. Refer to the "Sprouting Chart" for average time of maturation for each seed, bean or grain.

Sprouts will generally last as many days as it took for them to grow. For example, if the alfalfa sprouts took 7 days to grow, they will last 7 days.

Keep matured sprouts in the refrigerator. (The cold will slow down the growth of the sprouts, but won't stop it altogether.)
If you use the "jar" method, store the sprouts in a large glass jar or bowl, securely covered with cheesecloth and tipped at an angle so that any excess moisture can drain out.
If you use the "basket" method, you can put the basket with the sprouts and plastic all together in the refrigerator.
If you use the "bag" method, keep the bag, with the sprouts in it, in the refrigerator, and rinse it once every other day.


SPROUTING INGREDIENTS & EQUIPMENT

For both the "jar" and the "basket" method, you will need:

(1) Your choice of seeds, beans or grains. (For simplicity in giving directions, I am illustrating with alfalfa seeds.)
(2) One or two wide mouth jars, such as a mason jar, each 1 or 2 quart size.
(3) Cheese cloth or nylon mesh to cover the mouth of the jar.
(4) One or two rubber bands to secure the cheese cloth or mesh.

For the "basket" method, you will also need:

(5) An untreated straw basket (no shellac, please!) 9" wide, and 2 1/2" deep. Use one with a "tea-strainer" weave, which can usually be found at a houseware or oriental gift store.

(6) A plastic bag which fits over the basket and is strong enough not to "flop" onto the sprouts. (If you can't find one, you can order them from The Sprout House, New York City - see Bibliography, "Articles".)

The bag will create a "green house" effect. The plastic, unlike glass, will allow the sun's ultra violet rays to shine through the sprouts. Ultra violet rays are important for good health of the sprouts, and to kill any fungus.

(7) A gentle spray attachment for your faucet for rinsing the sprouts in the basket without disturbing their growth.

Don't be discouraged by the additional equipment required for the "basket" method. They are a one-time purchase, and well worth the advantages the "basket" method has.

For the "bag" method, you will need:

One or several flaxseed bags, 100% pure - no chemicals added. They can be ordered from The Sprout House, if you cannot find one in a store.

## DIRECTIONS FOR SPROUTING

### THE JAR METHOD
For Seeds, Beans or Grains

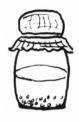
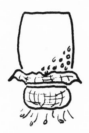
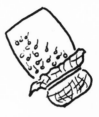
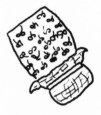

1.SOAK about 1 Tbl. alfalfa seeds for 4 hrs.

2. DRAIN off water

3.Set Jar at 45% angle. Rinse twice per day

4.Sprouts are ready in about 4 days. Refrigerate.

(1) Put one or two Tablespoons of the selected seeds (or 1 cup of grains or beans) into the jar. Cover with the mesh or cheesecloth, and secure with a rubber band.

(2) Rinse the seeds several times, then fill the jar half way with luke warm water, preferably spring water.

(3) Put the jar in a dark place, such as a cupboard. Let it soak overnight, or for the number of hours suggested on the "Sprouting Chart".

(4) After the soak time, drain off the excess water. Rinse the seeds thoroughly with lukewarm water, again draining off excess water.

(5) Rest the jar in a saucer or dish rack, open end down, at a 45% angle so that excess water can drain off and the sprouts can breathe. (See drawing #3.)

Be sure the mesh at the jar opening is not covered by sprouts or hulls, and that air is free to contact the sprouts. Occasionally you may need to remove the mesh and scoop off the hulls which often cling to the mesh.

Hulls will automatically separate from the seeds as they sprout. They can create rot, which spreads quickly and can spoil a whole batch of sprouts.

(6) Thoroughly rinse and drain the sprouts two to three times a day until they are ready to eat - usually 3 to 5 days. (See the "Sprouting Chart".) Don't let the seeds dry out. Keep them moist, but not too wet.

(7) After about 3 days, put vegetable sprouts, such as alfalfa, clover and radish sprouts, in the light to let them "green", which means that chlorophyll, so important for good health, is manufactured. (Bean and grain sprouts do not need to be "greened".)

To help prevent mold caused by rotting hulls, occasionally remove the hulls in the following way (especially before "greening" or refrigerating sprouts):

Put the sprouts in a large bowl of water. Swish them around gently. Some hulls will float to the top and some hulls will sink to the bottom. Scoop off the hulls that are on the surface of the water. Then remove the sprouts, being careful not to stir up the hulls at the bottom of the bowl.

## THE BASKET METHOD
### For seeds

To sprout in a basket, follow the "jar" method and directions for steps 1-4. Use 3 to 5 Tablespoons of seeds, depending on the size of your basket. (See p.110.) Then continue with the following steps:

(5) Pour the soaked seeds into your basket. Tip the basket at an angle for a few minutes to drain off any excess water. You can lean the basket on a towel.

(6) Put the basket of seeds into a plastic bag and tuck the bag loosely underneath, so that you have created a "greenhouse" effect, allowing a bubble of trapped air.

(7) Rinse the seeds twice a day, gently, but thoroughly, for a half a minute. Use a spray or shower adaptor, being careful not to disturb the root development. (The sprouts will ancor themselves by their roots to the weave of the basket.) Drain the basket well.

(8) When the hulls pop off and fall into the basket, rinse them off by immersing the basket in a basin of water. "Massage" the sprouts. The hulls will float up.
After a few days, when the roots are securely ancored, put the basket upside down in the water. Again, gently "massage" the sprouts, and the hulls will drop off.

(9) When the top layer of sprouts are mature, gently pull them out with your fingers, being careful not to disturb the young sprouts underneath. Give this new "generation" a day or two and they will "green up" and grow to maturity. After you pluck them, there will be a 3rd "generation", and perhaps even a fourth.

## THE BAG METHOD
For Grains and Beans

(1) Put about 1 cup grains or beans in a flaxseed bag. Soak the bag and seeds in pure water for 8 to 12 hours.

(2) Hang the bag up so it will drain.

(3) Rinse the bag twice a day in cold water. "Massage" the bag a little while rinsing, to help keep the sprouts from rooting themselves to the bag.

(4) The sprouts will be mature in 3 to 5 days. Refrigerate them, rinsing them once every other day.


## ADVANTAGES OF THE VARIOUS METHODS

### The Jar Method
The advantage in the "jar" method is that beans and grains, as well as seeds, can be sprouted in the jar.


### The Basket Method
For sprouting seeds, the "basket" method has several advantages over the "jar" method:

(1) The basket allows for vertical growth of these miniature vegetables. Greater surface area is exposed to the light, allowing for greater development of chlorophyll.

(2) Sprouts are generally longer and healthier.

(3) The "mature" sprouts can be "harvested" before the "immature" sprouts, so you can have 3 to 5 "generations" of sprouts. In other words, you will have a greater yield of mature, green sprouts (12 to 15 times their volume, compared with 7 to 8 times their volume when using a jar).

(4) It is easier to clean hulls off the sprouting seeds than with the "jar" method.

(5) There is less chance for spoilage.

## The Bag Method

For sprouting grains or beans, the bag method has several advantages over the jar method:

(1) The bags drain well, allowing the seeds to "breathe" freely.

(2) Flax fiber, which is the material of the bag, absorbs moisture, yet drains perfectly and maintains its coolness. For this reason, sprouts can be "watered" with a low risk of spoilage.

(3) Flax fiber is resistent to tearing, is light weight, easily transported, and takes up little space.

(4) The method of soaking and rinsing is simpler than with the jar method.

## CHART FOR SPROUTING.

(From "Recipes for Life" - Dr. Ann Wigmore)

| SEED. | SOAKING (Hours) | RINSING Times/day | READY IN (Days). |
|---|---|---|---|
| ADUKI | 8 - 12 | 3 | 3 - 5 |
| ALFALFA | 5 - 8 | 2 - 3 | 3 - 6 |
| CHICK PEAS | 8 - 15 | 4 | 3 - 4 |
| GARBANZO PEAS | 8 - 15 | 4 | 3 - 4 |
| CORN | 8 - 15 | 3 | 2 - 3 |
| FAVA BEANS ** | 8 - 12 | 3 | 3 - 4 |
| FENUGREEK | 6 - 8 | 3 | 3 - 4 |
| LENTILS | 8 - 12 | 3 | 2 - 3 |
| MILLET | 5 - 8 | 3 | 3 - 4 |
| MUNG BEANS | 8 - 12 | 4 | 5 - 6 |
| OATS | 5 - 8 | 2 | 3 - 4 |
| PEAS | 8 - 15 | 2 | 3 - 5 |
| RADISHES | 5 - 8 | 2 | 3 - 5 |
| RED CLOVER | 5 - 8 | 4 | 5 - 7 |
| RYE | 8 - 12 | 3 | 2 - 3 |
| SOY BEANS | 15- 24 | 4 | 3 - 4 |
| SUNFLOWER SEEDS | 8 | 2 | 24 hrs. |
| WHEAT | 8 - 15 | 2 | 2 - 3 |

" " " " " " " " " " " " " " " " " " " " " " " " " " " " " " " " " " " " " " " " " " " " "

** The same applies for all beans: black white, haricot, kidney, lima, navy, pinto, and red beans, etc...

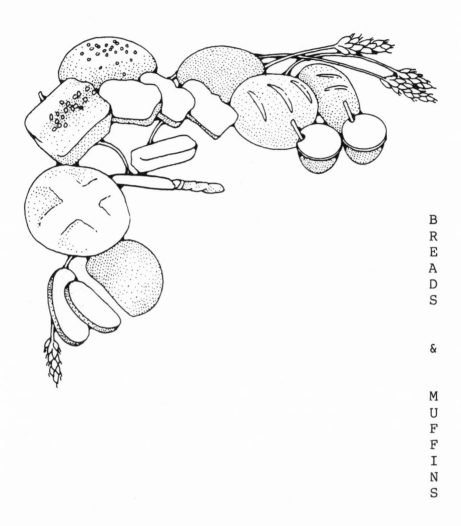

B
R
E
A
D
S

&

M
U
F
F
I
N
S

B R E A D S
******** &
M U F F I N S
********

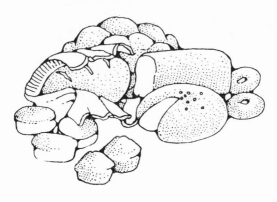

There are many marvelous recipe books that you can consult for baking a variety of delicious breads. The emphasis here is on breads that are easy to make and primarily wheat free.

Essene bread is a thick, chewy bread, made from sprouted grains and baked on a low heat. Because it is nearly raw, it is especially high in nutrients and vitality.

The Quick 2-Slice Bread Recipe was created out of the dilemma of wanting a slice of wheat-free bread for a meal or two, but not wanting to buy a whole loaf, or take the time to bake one. The recipe creates two slices of delicious bread that are done in 15 minutes and are sturdy enough to top with a spread and sprouts.

To help avoid an allergy to wheat, vary your grains as much as possible. (See "Allergens", Foods to Avoid, p.55.)

Since all flour should be refrigerated (See "Natural Food Kitchen Hints"), warm the amount of flour you need before using it for about 15 minutes on a low oven (150°). If you are using wheat germ, which is also refriger-ated, warm that, too.

******** BREAD RECIPES ********

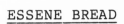

ESSENE BREAD

This bread is
raw, made from sprouted grains.

Use any of the following grains:
  wheat        unhulled barley        triticale
  rye          whole oats

Soak 1 1/2 c. grain overnight in 4 c. water.

In the morning, drain the water and let the grains sprout for 36 hours or more, until their "tails" measure about 1/8 inch long. During this time, rinse them 2-3 times a day.

Grind the sprouts in a hand grinder, seed processor, or champion juicer.
Kneed the sticky mixture until it is a dough-like consistency and it begins to hold shape.

Add any flavorings you like, such as:
chopped dates        chia seeds        sesame seeds
caraway seeds        garlic           dill seeds
sunflower seeds      onion            chives
raisins              cumin

Shape into loaves or patties. Lightly oil the surface of the dough and place on a well-oiled pan.
Put the pan in a low heat oven - 150°, or on a warm spot of a wood stove, or in the summer sun. The bread is done when there is a thin crust on the outside, and the inside is soft and moist, but not sticky. (Approximately 6 to 8 hours of drying.)
Note that this bread will be heavier than those to which you are accustomed.

## EVA'S BREAD

3 c. rye or whole wheat flour
1 Tbl. baking powder
1 1/2 c. water
3 Tbl. honey
2 eggs

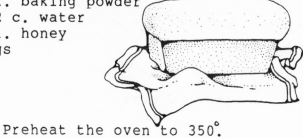

Preheat the oven to 350°.

Thoroughly mix the flour and baking powder. Blend the water, honey and eggs in a blender, then pour the mixture over the dry ingredients. Mix well, using quick strokes. Place in a lightly oiled or buttered loaf pan and bake at 350° for about 55 minutes, or until the top is well browned. Let it cool before slicing.

Variations:
Use any whole grain flour, such as millet, oat, barley, etc., or any combination of flours. (You may need to add more flour or water to get the same dough consistency.)
Add to the bread dough nuts or seeds, such as 2-3 tsp. caraway, sesame or sunflower seeds, or add raisins, chives, sliced onion or herbs. For a spice bread add more honey and/or molasses, plus cinnamon, ginger and allspice.
To make rolls, use 2 c. flour, 1 Tbl. powder, 2 egg, 2 Tbl. honey and 1 c. water. Bake in muffin tins at 325° for 30-35 minutes, until the tops are golden brown. This makes 8 muffins.
Experiment to your heart's content.

The bread recipe is from "The Good Book Cookbook" (See Bibliography).

## QUICK 2-SLICE BREAD

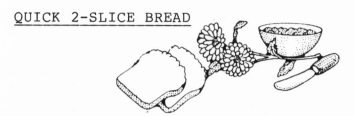

      If you have some left-over cereal, and wish you had a slice of bread, create two slices in your toaster oven in a manner of minutes. (See "Cereals" for cereal recipes.)

### Ingredients
    1/2 c. buckwheat porridge (or) creamy rice cereal, (or) cornmeal cereal cooked with almond milk as per the recipe.
    1/4 c. almonds
    1 egg

Grind the almonds in a blender. If you want some chunks of nuts in the bread, don't completely pulverize the nuts.
Leave the ground nuts in the blender. Add to the blender the cooked grain and one egg. Blend well.
Lightly grease your toaster oven pan. Spoon two large circles, or squares of the mixture onto the pan. Spread them out slightly so that they are a little flat, like bread.
Bake at 400°: 15 minutes for buckwheat bread, or 1/2 hour for corn or rice bread.

The buckwheat bread is delicious with 1 tsp. caraway seeds added to the batter. Top the bread with miso/tahini spread and alfalfa sprouts. (Also note that buckwheat porridge can be prepared very quickly. See recipe.)

Top the cornmeal bread with butter and honey.

Note: For a low-heat baking method, preheat the toaster oven to 450°. Put the bread in the oven. Turn the heat off. Let sit overnight.

MILLET BANANA BREAD (Makes 1 loaf)

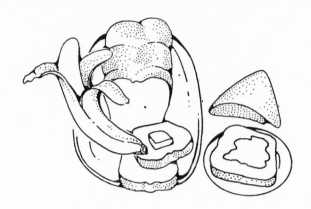

      1 c. mashed bananas (about 2 bananas)
      2 eggs, beaten
      1/4 c. honey
      1/4 c. melted butter (1/2 stick)
      2 Tbl. plain yogurt (optional)
      1 c. millet flour (purchased, or freshly
          ground in your nut-seed or grain
          grinder, or ex-coffee mill)
          1 tsp. baking soda
          1/2 c. chopped walnuts (optional)

Preheat the oven to 350°.

Mix the wet ingredients in one bowl, and the
dry ingredients in another bowl. Combine
them, then pour into a lightly greased 9x3x5"
loaf pan.
Bake at 350° for 55-60 minutes.

ZUCCHINI BREAD (Makes 1 loaf)

Preparation time: 35 minutes
Baking time: 45-55 minutes

    2 eggs, beaten
    2 Tbl. plain yogurt
    3/4 c. honey
    1/4 c. melted butter (1/2 stick)
    1 c. grated zucchini (about 1 medium sized
       zucchini)
    1 tsp. baking soda
    1 1/2 c. whole wheat pastry flour
    1 1/2 tsp. ground cinnamon
    1/2 c. chopped walnuts (optional)

Preheat the oven to 350°.

In a large bowl beat the eggs, then add the
yogurt and mix well. Add the melted butter
and honey and mix well, then add the grated
zucchini and mix well.
In a separate bowl, mix the dry ingredients.
Add the dry ingredients to the wet and mix
well.
Lightly grease a 9x5x3" loaf pan. Pour the
mixture into the pan and bake at 350° for
45-55 minutes. It's done when a toothpick
comes out clean in the center and the edges
are a medium brown. Gently remove and let
cool on a wire rack.


Note: To make a PUMPKIN SPICE BREAD, use
this same recipe with the following changes:
   Use 1 cup steamed, mashed pumpkin in place
of raw, grated zucchini.
   In addition to the cinnamon, use 1/2 tsp.
allspice, 1/8 tsp. nutmeg and 1/8 tsp.
ginger. Bake at 350° for 55 minutes.

## GINGERBREAD

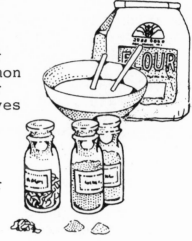

1 1/2 c. rice flour
1 c. oat flour
2 tsp. baking powder
1 tsp. ground cinnamon
1 tsp. ground ginger
1/4 tsp. ground cloves

3 egg yolks
1/2 c. molasses
3/4 c. honey
1/2 c. melted butter
1/4 c. water

3 egg whites

Preheat the oven to 350°.

Mix the flours, baking powder and spices in a large bowl.
In a medium sized bowl, beat the egg yolks. Add the melted butter, honey, molasses and water. Stir till well mixed.
Add the liquid ingredients to the dry, and stir till well blended.
In a medium sized bowl, beat the egg whites until they form soft peaks.
Fold the egg whites gently into the batter.
Pour into a lightly greased 8" baking pan.

Bake at 350° for 40-45 minutes, or until done. Gently remove the bread from the pan and let cool on a wire rack.

Top with pure whipped cream. (Sweetener is not necessary, although if you like, you could add a small amount of honey.)
Or, top with lemon frosting or kefir cheese.

## CORN MUFFINS

(Makes 16 muffins)

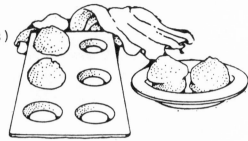

Preheat the oven to 425°, and lightly grease 16 muffin tins. Put a little water in any empty tins, to protect the tins.

Beat together in a bowl, or blend in a blender the following wet ingredients:

    3 egg
    6 Tbl. melted butter
    3 Tbl. honey
    1 3/4 c. water

Note: Before the butter has cooled, add the honey to it and stir until the honey dissolves. Add the water to this mixture to cool it off before adding it to the eggs. Otherwise, the hot butter may cook the eggs.

In a large bowl, mix together the following dry ingredients:

    3 c. cornmeal
    1 Tbl. baking powder (aluminum-free)
    optional: 1/2 tsp. sea salt

Add the wet ingredients to the dry, and stir till well mixed. Scoop or ladle the batter from the bottom of the mixing bowl (in case the cornmeal settles) and pour into each muffin mold, leaving some room for the dough to rise. Bake for 20 minutes at 425°, or until the muffins are golden brown.

APPLESAUCE MUFFINS (Makes 8 muffins)

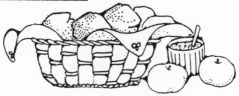

    3/4 c. ground rolled oats (Grind 1 c.
      rolled oats in your blender.)
    3/4 c. brown rice flour
    1 tsp. baking soda
    3 Tbl. honey
    1/4 c. melted butter
    1 egg yolk
    1/2 tsp. orange extract
    1 Tbl. grated organic orange peel
    3/4 c. unsweetened applesauce
    1/2 c. currants
    1 egg white

Preheat the oven to 400°.
Lightly grease an 8 cup muffin pan.

In a large mixing bowl, mix the ground rolled
oats, brown rice flour and baking soda.
In a smaller bowl, beat the egg yolk. Add the
honey, melted butter, orange extract and
grated orange peel. Stir well till mixed. Add
the applesauce and the currants, stirring
till mixed.
Slowly add the liquid ingredients to the dry,
stirring with quick strokes till combined.
Beat the egg white till it forms soft peaks.
Gently fold the beaten egg white into the
batter till well mixed.
Spoon the batter into the greased muffin
tins, filling them two-thirds full.
Bake at 400° for 20-25 minutes till done.
Remove the muffins from the tin and let cool
on a wire rack.

Variation:
Omit the orange extract and grated orange
peel. Add 1 tsp. cinnamon.

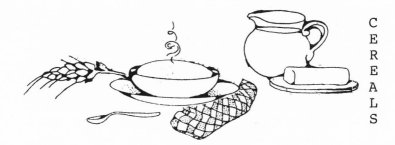

C
E
R
E
A
L
S

******** C E R E A L S ********

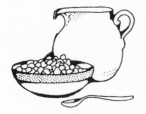
Cereals that are easy to pre-
pare, delicious and well
balanced proteins are a
wonderful way to start a day
and to sustain strength and
energy for hours.

## INGREDIENTS FOR CEREALS

### Whole Grains
        oats: rolled or sprouted.
        millet: whole, freshly ground,sprouted.
        barley: whole, freshly ground, roasted.
        rice: whole, freshly ground.
        rye: sprouted, flaked, freshly ground.
        buckwheat: unroasted or roasted (kasha).
        wheat: freshly ground or sprouted.
        corn meal.

### Nuts and Seeds
        soaked, freshly ground or sprouted:
        almonds              sunflower seeds
        sesame seeds         pumpkin seeds
        chia seeds           flax seeds
        caraway seeds

### Rehydrated (Soaked) Dried Fruit
        whole or chopped:
        prunes      raisins      apricots
        dates       figs

### Fresh Fruit
        bananas      peaches      apples

### Other Optional Cereal Ingredients
        grated coconut       butter
        honey                maple syrup
        barley malt          molasses
        soy sauce            cinnamon
        tahini               miso

        raw egg: stir into cereal

## LIQUID BASES OR TOPPINGS FOR CEREALS

Water
Nut/seed milk, soy milk or grain water (See
  "Beverages" for recipes.)
Juice, such as apple juice

Cereals can be cooked in, or topped with
these liquids.

### GENERAL CEREAL COOKING TECHNIQUES

Cereals, as with any grains, should be
cooked on low heats to preserve nutrients and
vitality. See "Grains" for detailed information on cooking grains and for a grain cooking chart.


Cereals can be cooked in any of the
following ways, depending on the type of
grain:

(1.) For rolled oats, buckwheat or
sprouted grain:
  Bring grain and liquid just to the boil,
shut off the heat, cover the pot and let the
grain cook in its own steam.

(2.) For any cooked grain:
  (a) In a blender, blend cooked grain
with hot liquid, or,
  (b) Heat the cooked grain in a pot with
a liquid, then eat as is, or blend.

(3.) For sprouted grain, whole or
ground brown rice, millet, barley or rye:
  (a) Gently cook on the lowest possible
heat, or,
  (b) Soak the grain for 24 to 36 hours.
Then, the night before eating the cereal,
bring the grain close to the boil, shut off
the heat, cover the pot and let the grain
cook in its own steam.

## HELPFUL CEREAL HINTS

### Time Saving Premix

Mix any of the following cereal ingredients in any combination(s) and keep them in glass jars in the freezer (to avoid rancidity) till use:

| | |
|---|---|
| nuts and seeds | grated coconut |
| dried fruit | whole grains |
| sprouted grain | |

### For Easier Digestibility:

Soak or grind the nut/seed mixture before adding to the cereal. Flax, sesame and chia, especially, should be ground since they are too small and hard to be chewed well.

Soak the dried fruit mixture over night, or add to the cereal before cooking.

### For A More Complete Protein:

Mix different kinds of grains, and add a variety of nuts and seeds to your cereals. For example, mix millet, wheatberries, buckwheat, and sesame, sunflower and flax seeds.
Or, use nut milk or soy milk to top your cereal, or as a cooking liquid.

### Flavor Changer:

Cook the cereal in nutmilk instead of water. Use different kinds of nuts and seeds and, in a blender, blend different sweeteners and/or dried fruit in the nutmilk.

******** CEREAL RECIPES ********

Cereal recipes are categorized by preparation time, since that is often an important consideration in the morning. The
categories are as follows:

"SUPER QUICK CEREALS": These take 10 to
20 minutes.

"30 MINUTE CEREALS": These take between
30 and 45 minutes, although with some planning ahead they can take less time without
sacrificing nutrition.

"THINK AHEAD CEREALS": These take some
pre-preparation, but once that is done, are
super quick and super delicious.


SUPER QUICK CEREALS

These take 10 to 20 minutes, including
preparation and cooking time.

OATMEAL (Makes 1 cup)

1/2 c. rolled oats
1 1/4 c. water or nut milk
Optional: 1-2 Tbl. raisins and/or honey

Put the water or nut milk in a pot. Add the
oats (and dried fruit). Bring the liquid
close to a boil while stirring.
Turn the heat off, cover the pot, and let the
oatmeal cook in its own steam till soft
(about 10 minutes).
Eat as is, or add butter and/or soy or nut
milk, or tahini and/or miso.

Or, put the cooked oatmeal through the
blender with hot water or nut milk and eat it
creamy.

BUCKWHEAT PORRIDGE (Makes 1 cup)

(Note: Buckwheat is not wheat. Those with wheat allergies can often tolerate buckwheat.)

1/2 c. buckwheat or kasha (roasted buckwheat)
1/2 c. water

Put the buckwheat and water in a pot. Bring the water just to the boil. Turn off the heat. Stir the buckwheat with a fork. Cover the pot and let sit till soft (5-10 minutes). Top with nut milk, or butter and soy sauce. (This makes a great side dish, as well.)

Optional: Add soaked dried fruit.


QUICK CREAM OF GRAIN CEREAL (Makes 1 cup)

2 Versions:

1.  Grind nuts and seeds in a dry blender. Add about 3/4 c. cooked grain (such as brown rice or millet) and 1/4 c. hot water. Blend again. Add as much water as you like for the consistency desired.
                        (or)

2.  Warm cooked grain in a pot with almond or soy milk. Eat as is or blenderize.

For optional additions, see pp.130-131.

For a less sweet taste that is delicious, try re-heating or blending the cooked grain in soy milk and a pinch of cinnamon. Or, in place of cinnamon, add a small amount of light miso when the cereal is ready to eat.

Note: Adding nuts and seeds, nut milk or soy milk to cereals not only enhances the flavor, but increases the utilizable protein.

## 30-MINUTE CEREALS

### 30 MINUTE CREAM OF GRAIN CEREAL(Makes 1 c.)

1/4 c. freshly ground brown rice or millet

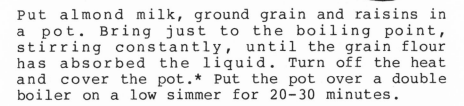

1 c. almond milk (See p.156.)
Sweeten the almond milk with
honey or molasses, cinnamon,
and pure vanilla extract.
1/4 c. raisins

Put almond milk, ground grain and raisins in
a pot. Bring just to the boiling point,
stirring constantly, until the grain flour
has absorbed the liquid. Turn off the heat
and cover the pot.* Put the pot over a double
boiler on a low simmer for 20-30 minutes.

* Note: For quicker cooking in the morning,
prepare the grain up to this point the night
before, soaking the grain and the raisins in
the hot liquid overnight. In the morning,
bring it close to the boil again, then put it
over the double boiler for 10 to 15 minutes.

Optional: Add sliced bananas and/or nut milk.


### MILLET CEREAL (Makes 1 cup)

1/4 c. millet        1 c. water or nut milk
Optional: nuts/seeds or dried fruit

Put the water or nut milk (plus optional ex-
tras) in a pot. Bring just to the boil, then
turn heat down to the lowest possible setting. Cook about 20 minutes, till soft. Eat
as is, or with sliced bananas and nut milk.

## CORN MEAL CREAM CEREAL (Makes 1 1/2 c)

(Takes about 45 minutes, including cooking)

1 1/4 c. almond milk
1 tsp. molasses
1/4 - 1/2 tsp. cinnamon     1/8 tsp. vanilla
1/4 c. corn meal         1 Tbl. raisins

Prepare the nut milk, blending into it the molasses, cinnamon and vanilla.
Meanwhile, heat water in the bottom of a double boiler, leaving it at a low simmer.

Put the nut milk in the top of the double boiler. Put that pot directly over the burner and while bringing the nut milk close to a boil, slowly pour in the corn meal (plus raisins) while stirring constantly with a wire whisk to avoid lumping.
When the almond milk has absorbed the corn meal, cover the pot and put it over the bottom of the double boiler.
Let stand over the double boiler, which is still at a low simmer, 1/2 hour.

## BROWN BARLEY CREAM CEREAL (Makes 1 cup)

1/4 c. barley 3/4 c. water
1 tsp. raw honey

Spread the barley kernels thinly in a frying pan. Brown them lightly, stirring constantly. (This procedure is not necessary, but makes a more delicious taste.)
Put the browned barley in a pot. Add the water. Bring just to the boiling point. Take the pot off the heat. Cover and let stand 20 minutes.
If you like, blend the cooked barley, adding honey, barley malt, miso or molasses, etc. Top with nut milk.

## THINK AHEAD CEREALS

These cereals take some thinking ahead and pre-paration, but are well worth it! (This could also include the super quick rice, millet and barley cream cereals since the grains must be cooked ahead of time.)

### SPROUTED CEREAL: WHEAT OR RYE

(See section on "Sprouts".)
1 ounce of dry seed produces about 1 cup of mature sprouts. Sprouts can expand to at least 8 times their seed size.

To use sprouted grains as a cereal, mix them in any combination you like by themselves or with the quick-cook grains (such as rolled oats, rye flakes, buckwheat, etc.) Add freshly ground or soaked nuts and seeds, soaked dried fruit, etc. Top with nut milk.

### THERMOS CEREAL

For any grain except wheat, which comes out "rubbery". The rolled or flaked cereals, also, may be too "mushy" cooked this way.
See "Grains" for more details.

Use a 1 quart <u>wide mouthed</u> thermos. Add the grain and any other ingredients (nuts and seeds, dried fruit, etc.), then the required amount of liquid, brought close to a boil. (Do not fill water right up to the top. Allow at least 1 inch from the top.)
Screw the lid on tightly and let stand 8 to 12 hours.
Grains can be put into the thermos whole or ground. If you like, blend the cooked cereal.

## SUPER CEREAL

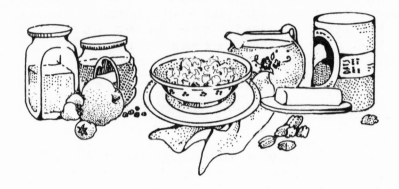

### Step 1.
Put a mixture of grains in a large bowl or jar and add water 2 1/2 times the volume of the grain. Let stand on the counter for 36 hours at room temperature.

### Step 2.
After the 36 hour soaking time, refrigerate. To keep it fresh and moist, cover the grain with water. This will keep for several days.

### Step 3.
The night before you want the cereal, remove 1/2 to 1 cup of the mixture, leaving the remaining portion covered with water in the refrigerator.
Put the 1/2 to 1 cup pre-soaked mixture in a pot, add any additional quick-cook grains, nuts and seeds, dried fruit, plus an equal amount of water.
Bring the water just to the boil, shut the heat off, cover the pot, and let stand over-night.

Step 4.
The next morning, warm the mixture, and add to taste: honey or barley malt, butter, and nut or soy milk.


Suggested Grains to Pre-soak
brown rice                    millet
wheatberries                  whole rye

Add the night before
rye flakes          rolled oats          buckwheat
sunflower seeds   pumpkin seeds        almonds
dried fruit  shredded coconut
ground flax and/or sesame seeds

Note: All ingredients listed under "Add the night before" can be pre-mixed to taste and kept on hand in the freezer.

GOLDEN ROASTED GRANOLA (Makes about 5 cups)

    1/4 c. melted butter
    1/4 c. honey or barley malt
    1 tsp. vanilla extract
    3 c. rolled oats
    1 tsp. cinnamon
    3 oz. hulled, ground
        sesame seeds
    3/4 c. dry roasted,
        unsalted soybeans
    3/4 c. chopped almonds,
        pecans or walnuts
    3 oz. ground flax seeds
Optional: 1 c. shredded coconut or 3/4 c.
    dates; 1 c. raisins

    Preheat oven to 250°. Mix the butter, honey
or barley malt, and vanilla. Mix the oats and
cinnamon in another bowl. Pour the butter
mixture over the oat mixture and mix well.
    Lightly oil a flat pan. Thinly spread the
mixture onto the pan.
    Bake for 1 to 1 1/2 hours, stirring
occasionally, until the mixture is a light
golden brown. (For lower-heat baking, preheat
the oven to 300° the night before, then shut
it off when you put the pan in, and leave it
overnight.)
    Remove the mixture from the oven, and add
the nuts and seeds and any optional
ingredients. Store in an airtight container
in the refrigerator.

    Note: The dry ingredients can be pre-
mixed and kept in jars in the freezer till
use.

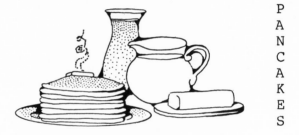

P
A
N
C
A
K
E
S

*********** P A N C A K E S **********

## GENERAL PANCAKE COOKING HINTS

To test your griddle to see if it is the right heat, drop a little water on it. If the water bounces around, the griddle is the right heat. If the water just sits there, it is not hot enough. If the water quickly evaporates, the griddle is too hot.

Spoon the pancake batter onto the griddle from a height just above the pan. The pancake will be ready to turn when tiny air bubbles form (and before they pop). Usually the pancake will take half the cooking time on the other side, after it is turned.

To keep the pancakes warm, put them on a baking sheet in a low oven. Do not stack them right on top of each other, or they will get rubbery. Put a cloth between each one.

RECIPES

BUCKWHEAT PANCAKES (about 2 dozen)
    1 c. buckwheat flour
    1/2 c. brown rice flour
    1/2 tsp. baking soda
    1 1/2 c. buttermilk
    4 Tbl. butter, melted
    2 eggs, beaten

Combine the flours and the baking soda.
In a separate bowl, beat the eggs. Add the melted butter and buttermilk.
Add the liquid ingredients to the dry, combining them well with quick strokes. Add water till you have a fairly runny batter. (About 1/3 to 1/2 c. water.)

-142-

## CORNMEAL PANCAKES

    1 c. yellow cornmeal
    1 1/4 c. boiling water
    1/2 c. brown rice flour
    2 tsp. baking powder
    1 egg yolk
    1/2 c. almond milk (10 almonds ground, then
      blended with 1/2 c. water and 2 tsp.
      honey.)
    2 Tbl. melted butter
    1 egg white

    Put the cornmeal in a large bowl. Slowly stir in the 1 1/4 c. boiling water till well combined. Let stand 10 minutes.

    In a separate bowl, beat the egg yolk. Add the almond milk and butter.

    Combine the rice flour and baking powder, then add to the cornmeal.

    Add the liquid ingredients and stir till well mixed.

    Beat the egg white till it forms soft peaks. Gently fold the beaten egg white into the batter.

    If necessary, add more water so that the batter is slightly runny.

## PANCAKE VARIATIONS

    Add to pancake batter any of the following:

| | |
|---|---|
| chopped banana | chopped walnuts |
| blueberries | chopped apples |
| ground cinnamon | |

FOR PANCAKE TOPPINGS, SEE NEXT PAGE.

PANCAKE TOPPINGS

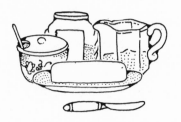

Pancakes are great topped with any of the following:

* pure maple syrup

* homemade mixtures, such as:
  honey + butter + cinnamon
                (or)
  barley malt + butter + cinnamon
                (or)
  molasses + butter + cinnamon
                (or)
  tahini, barley malt, cinnamon, and water, mixed well to thin

* fresh fruit jam or marmalade, such as honey carrot marmalade or strawberry jam, p.212.

* applesauce, p.290.

* yogurt or kefir cheese

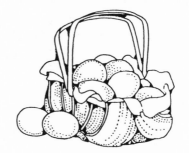

E
G
G
S

*******  E G G S  *******

Soft boiling or poaching eggs are the best ways to cook eggs, since overcooked proteins are less utilizable by the body and are often difficult to digest.[1.]

## SOFT BOILING

Put the egg(s) in a pot and cover with cool water. Bring the water close to a boil, then turn the heat off. Let the egg(s) cook in the steam water, covered, for 2-4 minutes, depending on how "runny" you like them.

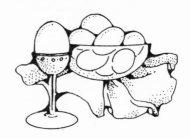

## OMELETTES

If you make omelettes, cook with a small amount of butter or olive oil on the lowest possible heat, and do not over-cook it.

A delicious omelette filling :
plain yogurt
chopped scallion
alfalfa sprouts
sliced zucchini, raw or lightly steamed

(or)
cottage cheese
sliced avocado
chopped watercress leaves

## SCRAMBLING AND FRYING

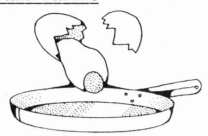

If you scramble or fry your eggs, do it in a small amount of butter or olive oil on a low heat. Alfalfa sprouts are delicious added to scrambled eggs after cooking.

## POACHING

Bring about 2" water in a fry pan to a low simmer; i.e., below the boiling point. Add a drop of apple cider vinegar. (This helps hold the egg together.)

Crack one egg at a time, slipping it into the gently simmering water. If the white of the egg spreads too far, you can gently push it toward the yolk with a spatula. Simmer for 4 to 5 minutes, or remove the pan from the heat and let sit 8 minutes. Cook the egg till it holds, but is not hard.

Some people find that the egg will be less likely to spread if they make a whirlpool in the water with a spoon before adding the egg. Then slip the egg into the center of the well of the whirlpool.

If there are streamers of white after the egg is cooked, you can cut them off with scissors before serving.

If you have difficulty digesting proteins and starches together, so that you cannot have poached eggs on toast, try it over steamed broccoli. Put a small amount of butter and/or lemon juice on the broccoli, before adding the egg.

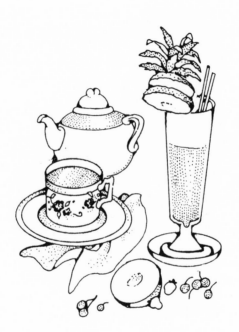

B
E
V
E
R
A
G
E
S

******** B E V E R A G E S ********

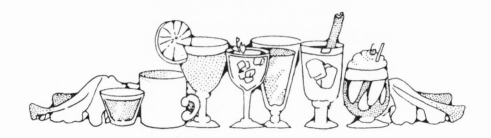

Fresh juices and blender drinks made from raw vegetables and fruits, nuts and seeds and grains are perhaps the most delicious and enjoyable way to fill an undernourished body with a concentration of quickly and easily assimilated nutrients, while gently, but powerfully accelerating the process of detoxification and regeneration.

Juices and blender drinks are a great way to get a lot of variety in the diet.

Freshly juiced vegetables, greens and fruits can also be used effectively, under your doctors care, to lose or gain weight, or to undertake a health regaining juice fast.

Juices and blender drinks can also provide crucial nourishment to those with denture problems or extreme digestive stress.

In addition, when you have more fruits, vegetables and leafy greens than you can use in your recipes, they need not go to waste. Juice or blend them in any of the delicious combinations suggested in this recipe section.

## BEVERAGE VARIETIES

Delicious and healthful beverages can be prepared quickly and easily with a juice extractor or a blender, depending on the recipe, and there is an almost unlimited variety:

## NUT SEED MILKS

Nut-Seed milks are "milky" liquids made by blending nuts and seeds, or nut/seed butters (such as tahini or almond butter), and water. They are a good source of easily assimilated protein, of B vitamins and other vitamins, minerals, oils and unsaturated fatty acids, and, best of all, they taste wonderful!

In a whole state, nuts and seeds can be difficult to chew, especially the smaller seeds, and are tempting to over-eat, a strain on the digestion and on over-weight. With nut milks, the nuts and seeds are broken down to a more easily digested form, and, since they are measured out in the preparation, the temptation to over indulge is eliminated.

Nut milks are a great substitute for cow's milk in any recipe, especially over cereal. They are non mucous forming, rarely allergenic, and provide calcium and other minerals necessary for calcium absorption and utilization. Sesame milk, especially, made with 2 Tbl. sesame seeds in 1 cup water, contains twice as much calcium as an equal amount of cow's milk, as well as a higher quality protein than a pound of meat.

Nut milks are also a wonderful base for smoothies and for beverages that provide a breakfast in a glass. Simply blend the nut milk with fruit, such as a banana or a raw egg to create the effect you desire.

## GRAIN WATER

For those who prefer not to have nuts and seeds or dairy, and/or need a large intake of minerals, grain water is an ideal solution.

It is delicious on cereals, as a snack, as a soup or sauce base, and is perfect for convalescing or denture problems. It is made by blending a small amount of cooked grain, such as barley, rice or millet with water.

Rejuvelac, or "fermented grain water", made by soaking wheat or rye berries in water for 24-48 hours, is an excellent source of lactic acid (which feeds "friendly bacteria", so necessary for a healthy colon), and of enzymes, and vitamins E and B.

## VEGETABLE COCKTAILS

Freshly juiced raw vegetables contain valuable vitamins, minerals, enzymes and natural sugars, and are easily digested since the cellulose has been removed. They can be prepared in many delicious combinations, according to taste preference and nutritional needs.

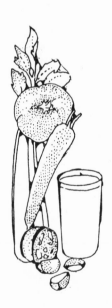

## GREEN DRINKS

Green drinks are a great way to get lots of chlorophyll, which is one of our most powerful aids in balancing, cleansing and rebuilding a weak body. Use a variety of greens, such as watercress, parsley, Romaine lettuce, etc. (See "recipe").

Wheatgrass juice, the juice from the green grass grown from wheat berries, is possibly the best source of chlorophyll we have. Simply chew the grass and spit out the pulp, or juice it with a press-type juicer designed to extract juice from wheatgrass. (Drink very small amounts of wheatgrass juice at a time, as it is very strong - not more than 1/2 - 1 oz.)

For sources for wheatgrass juicers, lists of equipment and instructions for growing wheatgrass, see footnote.[1]

## PINEAPPLE COCKTAILS

Pineapple juice combines well with vegetables and/or proteins, can aid the digestion, and has a gently cleansing action.

## OTHER JUICED AND BLENDED FRUITS

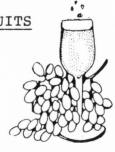

Children, and the child in each of us, especially love fruit juices in homemade soft drinks, in smoothies and in shakes.

******** BEVERAGE RECIPES ********

### NUT SEED MILKS

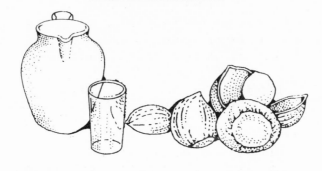

There are many variations on nut milks. Use your imagination and taste preferences to experiment.

For the value of "nut milks" see p.151.

## NUT SEED CHOICES

| | | |
|---|---|---|
| almond | sunflower | pumpkin |
| sesame | chia | flax |

Keep your own special mixture of whole nuts and seeds in a glass jar in the freezer (to avoid rancidity) to grind when needed. They take only seconds to grind.

Note that the "butters" made from nuts and seeds, such as tahini (sesame seed butter), or almond butter, can also be blended with water to form nut milks.

## LIQUID BASE VARIATIONS FOR NUT MILKS

water
pineapple juice       vegetable juice
grain water           soup bouillon

## NUT MILK BLENDING VARIATIONS

(1.) Soak nuts and seeds of your choice overnight, then blend with the liquid.
(or)
(2.) Without soaking first,:
    (a) Grind the nuts and seeds in a dry blender, then add liquid, or,
    (b) Put the nuts and seeds and liquid in the blender together, then blend.
(or)
(3) Blend tahini or almond butter with water.

The method of grinding the nuts and seeds depends on the type of blender, -- the strength and position of the blade. Find the method that works best for you.
A nut/seed grinder (your ex-coffee mill) works best for smaller seeds, such as sesame, flax, or chia. After grinding them, transfer them to the blender to blend with the liquid.
A normal blender or cuisinart will usually grind nuts and larger seeds, and sometimes larger quantities of smaller seeds.
You may wish to strain the nut milk after blending, to remove small particles, especially if you are feeding a small child.

## ADD TO NUT MILKS ANY OF THE FOLLOWING:

| | | |
|---|---|---|
| whey powder | soy powder | wheat germ |
| brewers yeast | raw egg | tofu |
| rice polishings | lemon juice | bran |
| tahini | almond butter | honey |
| molasses | barley malt | maple syrup |
| rice bran syrup | cinnamon | nutmeg |
| ground cloves | shredded coconut | |

black cherry concentrate
unsweetened carob powder (a "chocolate"taste)
cafix (a "coffee" flavor)
vanilla or almond extract
fresh or rehydrated (soaked) dried fruit
raw vegetables and/or leafy greens

## NUT MILK RECIPES

### Almond Milk (Makes 1 cup)

        8-10 almonds          3/4 c. water
        1/8 tsp. vanilla      1/4 tsp. honey

Grind the almonds in a dry blender, then add the water, vanilla and honey and blend well again. Strain, if necessary.

Optional: Some people prefer to blanch the almonds first; that is, to remove the skins.

Blanching almonds:
    Bring some water to a boil, drop the almonds in the water, turn the heat off and let the almonds sit a minute or two. Break a tiny hole in the skin of the pointed end of the almond, then squeeze the almond out of its skin into your other hand.

### SUNFLOWER ALMOND MILK (Makes 4 cups)

        1/4 c. sunflower seeds    3 c. water
        1/4 c. almonds            1 tsp. honey.

Grind the nuts and seeds in a dry blender. Add the honey and water. Blend again.

### SESAME MILK (Makes 1 cup)

        2 Tbl. sesame seeds or 1 1/2 Tbl. tahini
        1 c. water
        1/4 tsp. honey

Grind the sesame seeds. Then, in a blender, blend the ground seeds, water and honey. (If necessary, grind the seeds in a nut-seed grinder, then transfer to blender.)

## RECIPES FOR "BREAKFAST IN A GLASS"

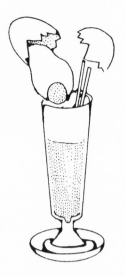

### SUNFLOWER-EGG

2 tsp. ground of each:
sunflower seeds
almonds

Blend well with:
1 raw egg
1 c. water

Optional: add 1 tsp. carob powder, 1 tsp.
vanilla and 1 tsp. honey.

### CHERRY EGG

1 tsp. ground of each:

sunflower seeds      flax seeds
sesame seeds         almonds
pumpkin seeds        chia seeds

Blend well with:
1 raw egg            1 1/2 c. water
1 tsp. black cherry concentrate

Optional: Add 1/2 banana

### EGG NOG (Serves 1)

For a dairy free egg nog, blend a raw
egg and a pinch of nutmeg in the basic almond
milk.

See recipes for PROTEIN PUNCH and PINEAPPLE
GREEN DRINK for other "BREAKFASTS IN A GLASS"

## SMOOTHIES AND SHAKES

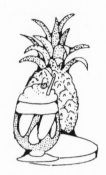

The combinations for
smoothies are unlimited.
Refer to "Blending Magic"
by Dr. Bernard Jensen,
for a wealth of recipes.
Here are a few good
combinations to blend
in your blender:

        1/2 banana + 1/2 c. pineapple juice
        1/2 banana + 1/2 c. coconut juice
                    and 1/4 c. pineapple juice
        1/2 banana + 1/2 c. apple juice

Use any fruits, nuts and seeds, nut milks, or
fruit juices in any combinations. Sliced
fresh fruit, such as mango or papaya, blended
with water is delicious by itself as a
smoothie, or put the mixture in a popsickle
mold and freeze it.

## BANANA SHAKE

        1 ripe, peeled banana
        1 c. almond milk (see "Nut Milk"), or
                        1 c. water + 1 Tbl. tahini
        1/4 tsp. honey.

Blend well in a blender.

VARIATIONS:
For a carob shake, add to the banana shake 1
Tbl. unsweetened carob powder and more honey
to taste.
For a mocha shake, add to the carob shake
1 tsp. cafix.
Whey powder can be added to the carob or
mocha shake.

BANAN-ALMOND FIG SHAKE

In a blender, blend till creamy:
    1/2 c. almond milk (See p.156.)
    1 ripe peeled banana
    2 black mission figs, soaked overnight,
              then chopped.
    1 tsp. rice polishings


TOFU MALT

Blend in a blender:
    1/4 c. ground almonds    1 Tbl. honey
    1/4 c. water             1/4 c. tofu
    1 Tbl. unsweetened carob powder


FENUGREEK FLUFF

    1/4 c. fenugreek seeds
    2 c. water and/or pineapple juice

Soak the seeds in the liquid all day. That night, blend the seeds and liquid together. Let the mixture sit overnight. If your blender is strong enough, blend the mixture again the next morning. If not, refrigerate as is. This is your stock. It should be quite thick and smooth. Do not be concerned if the stock is not very smooth, as you will be blending it again. The stock will keep, refrigerated, for several days in a closed glass or porcelain container.

To 1/4 c. stock, add and blend well in a blender 1 c. water or juice, and any of the following for flavor and nutritional variety:
    unsweetened carob powder
    pure vanilla or almond extract
    fresh fruit: rasberries, peaches, pa-
      paya, banana, blueberries, etc.

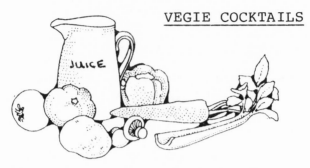

## VEGIE COCKTAILS

Vegetables can be juiced, or can be blended in a liquid (especially in the case of leafy greens).

### VEGETABLES TO JUICE

| | | |
|---|---|---|
| carrots | celery | beets |
| cabbage | potatoes | turnips |
| parsnips | cucumbers | tomatoes |

These vegetables are better juiced for a vegie cocktail. Blending them will make a raw soup (see "Soups").

### LEAFY GREENS TO JUICE, OR BLEND IN BLENDER

| | | |
|---|---|---|
| comfrey | parsley | basil |
| kale | spinach | wheatgrass |
| turnip greens | swiss chard | watercress |
| rugala | sorrel | dill |
| dandelion greens | romaine lettuce | |

Leafy greens can be juiced, or can be blended very well in a liquid such as pineapple juice, or a special herb tea, such as peach leaf, rasberry leaf or oatstraw.

### OPTIONAL VEGETABLE COCKTAIL ADDITIONS

freshly squeezed lemon or lime juice
minced garlic or onion
kelp or salt-free vegetable powder

## RECIPES FOR VEGIE COCKTAILS

### SUGGESTED COMBINATIONS TO JUICE

      carrot, celery, beet
      carrot, celery, beet, parsley
      fresh ginger, carrot
      cabbage, celery, parsley
      potato, beet
      carrot, apple

Please note: When using beet, do not use a beet larger than the size of a golf ball per person. It is heavily cleansing, and too much beet juice can cause unpleasant detoxification reactions. (Beets can also turn your eliminations red.) This is also true of certain bitter greens, such as watercress. Use only a small handful at a time. Mother Nature protects us by making such foods too bitter to overeat. Keep that in mind when juicing.

### MIXED VEGETABLE JUICE (Makes 2 c.)

1/2 c. carrot juice          1/2 c. celery juice
2 tsp. chopped parsley       1 c. tomato juice
1 tsp. lemon juice           1/8 tsp. basil
powdered kelp or dulse to taste

Mix well.

### BRILLIANT MARY (Serves 1)

8 oz. tomato juice           juice of 1/2 lemon
pinch  or more of cayenne pepper
1 clove finely minced garlic

Optional: add 1 oz. celery juice; 1 tsp. soy sauce; or, 1/2 tsp. horseradish.

## PINEAPPLE COCKTAILS

PROTEIN PUNCH (Makes 1 3/4 c.)

Soak 1 tsp. of the following overnight in pineapple juice:

| | |
|---|---|
| almonds | sunflower seeds |
| chia seeds | pumpkin seeds |
| flax seeds | sesame seeds |

In the morning, blend well, in a blender, with 1 1/2 c. of any of the following liquids:

water, or water and pineapple juice
pineapple juice
chamomile, oatstraw or rasberry leaf tea

## PINEAPPLE GREEN DRINK

To 1 c. pineapple juice (or 1/2 cup each of pineapple juice and water, if you prefer it a little less sweet) add and blend well, in a blender, the following:

1-2 sprigs watercress
1 handful parsley
1 large leaf romaine lettuce
1 large spinach leaf

Add more liquid, if necessary. If available, add 1 large leaf fresh comfrey, and/ or, 2 small leaves fresh basil or mint.

Optional: add 1 raw egg, and/ or, some nuts and seeds, such as the "Protein Punch" mixture.

## PINEAPPLE DRINK VARIATIONS

(Also see "Smoothies")

In a blender, blend 1 cup pineapple juice
with any of the following:
        1 raw egg and/ or 1/2 - 1 banana
        1 c. apple juice and 1 banana
        1 c. coconut water and 1 c. papaya juice
        1/2 c. fresh carrot juice and 1 tsp.
                        lemon juice
        ground nuts and seeds
        fresh or frozen strawberries

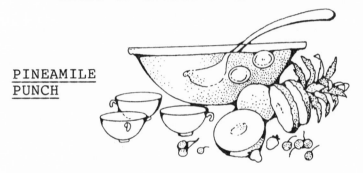

PINEAMILE
PUNCH

(This recipe is Thanks to Eva Graf)

        1 tsp. chamomile flowers
        1 c. water, brought to the boil
        1 tsp. honey, or more to taste
        1 c. pineapple juice

Pour the water over the chamomile flowers.
Steep 15 minutes, then strain. Add honey. Let
cool, then mix with pineapple juice.
This is delicious hot or cold.

PUNCH ALTERNATIVES AND VARIATIONS:
        Use papaya juice instead of pineapple
juice.
        Add spearmint or peppermint leaves when
steeping the tea.
        Add one whole clove and/or a pinch of
cinnamon when steeping.

## OTHER JUICED FRUITS

### HOT MULLED JUICE

To 1 quart apple cider
or pineapple juice add:
    2 cinnamon sticks
    4-5 cloves
    pinch ground nutmeg
    pinch allspice
    Opt: lemon juice to taste.

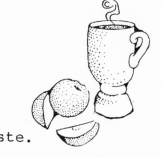

Bring the juice and spices close to the boil,
then turn the heat down to the lowest possible setting. Use a flame tamer, if possible.
Cover the pot. Let simmer 20 minutes.

### CRANBERRY JUICE
(This recipe thanks to Eva Graf)

    1 lb. cranberries
    2 qts.water
    1 tsp. freshly squeezed lemon juice
    honey to taste

Put the cranberries and water in a large soup
pot (2-3 qt. capacity). Place over a medium
hot stove.
As soon as bubbles begin to form, cover the
pot and take off the stove. Do not allow to
boil. (Boiling cranberries releases oxalic
acid which can be detrimental in excess.)
Let the cranberries sit, covered, for 25
minutes.
Separate most of the juice from the berries
and put the juice aside.
Blend the berries and a little juice. Strain
the mixture, throwing away the pulp.
Combine the strained mixture and the juice,
and add honey to taste.

## SPECIAL SOFT DRINKS

### FRUIT FIZZ

Mix chilled mineral
water or salt-free
seltzer water with
an equal amount of
fruit juice, such
as apple, pineapple,
grape or cranberry.
Or, Stir 1 tsp. of
pure fruit concentrate,
such as black cherry
concentrate, into 1 cup
of the fizzy water.

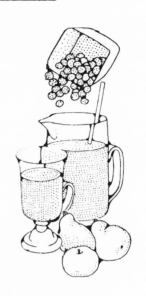

### HERBAL GINGER ALE

     1/4 tsp. powdered ginger
     1/4 c. hot water
     1/4 tsp. (more or less) honey
     1 small bottle chilled mineral water

Steep the ginger in the hot water for 10
minutes. Add the honey. Let cool, then add
the mineral water.

## GRAIN WATER RECIPES

For the value of "grain water", see p.152.

### BARLEY WATER

(Note that other grains, such as rice, rye or millet can also be used, by themselves or in combinations.)

1 Tbl. uncooked barley          2 c. water
Opt: Add raw honey, barley malt or molasses to taste after blending.

Cook the grain in the water as per Low Heat Cooking Techniques under "Grains" (See p. 245.). Or, bring the water close to the boil, turn the heat down to the lowest possible setting, cover the pot and let simmer 1/2 hour. Then, in a blender, blend the grain in the water very well and, if you like, strain the remaining grain pieces out.

Opt: For a different taste, before cooking the grain, lightly roast it in a dry pan.

### GRAIN WATER VARIATION

For a variety in nourish-ment, blend into the grain water raw greens or vege-tables. If necessary, strain. For example, in a blender, blend raw kale or parsley and barley water.

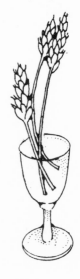

_____

## REJUVELAC (Fermented Grain Water)

For the value of "rejuvelac", see p.152.

1 c. soft pastry wheat berries, rye berries
    or barley
3 c. water

Wash the grain by rinsing it well. Allow dead
seeds to float to the top, and remove them.
Put the grain in a large bowl. Cover with the
3 c. water. Allow enough room at the top of
the bowl for the grain to expand and the
water level to rise about 4". Put a clean
cloth over the bowl and let it sit for 24 to
48 hours. (If you like a tangy taste, 48
hours is better.)
After the allowed soaking time, drain the
fermented grain water into a pitcher, keeping
the grain in the first bowl. Add 2 more cups
of water to the grain and let sit another 24
hours.
After the second 24 hours, drain the
fermented water into the first batch of
fermented grain water, combining them.
If you like, soak the berries a third time
and combine with the other batch.
If the berries are not too glutenous, you can
grind them for cereal or for raw bread.

HERB TEAS

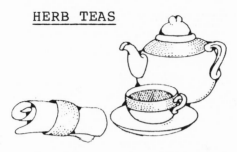

There is as much variety in herb teas as there is in plants and spices. Experiment to find the one you most enjoy.

PREPARING HERB TEAS

For Leaves and Flowers:
Put the herb in a tea pot or in a cup. In a saucepan or tea kettle, bring the water just to the boil, then pour over the herb.
Cover the pot or cup and and let the herb steep 10-20 minutes.

For roots and pits:
Bring the water and the herb just to the boil, then turn the heat down to the lowest possible heat and let simmer 20 minutes.

Use approximately 1 tsp. dried herb per cup of water.
Pour the herb tea into a cup through a non-aluminum strainer.
Add honey, if you like.

Note that herb teas can also be used as a base for a blender drink or for cooking grains as a way of providing additional nutritional support and boosting flavor.

## HERB TEA RECIPES

### MINT REFRESHER

To 8 oz. peppermint or spearmint tea, add 1
tsp. honey and 1 tsp. lemon juice.
For a summer refresher, make the tea extra
strong, add more honey, let cool, then add
ice cubes.

### SPECIAL CALCIUM TEA

       1 tsp. chamomile flowers
       1 tsp. oatstraw
       1 tsp. dried comfrey
       1 tsp. alfalfa
       2 c. water

Put the herbs in a pot. Bring the water just
to the boil. Pour the water over the herbs,
cover the pot, and let steep 20 minutes.

### TUMMY SOOTHER

Mix together the following:
       1 tsp. dried peppermint leaves
       1 tsp. dried chamomile flowers
       1 tsp. dried ground fennel

Steep in 2 c. water.
Add 1/2 tsp. honey.
Let cool, then add 1/4 c. papaya juice, or 1
Tbl. fresh papaya blended in water.

This tea has a light licorice taste.

## SPECIAL LIQUID TREATS

### HONIGAR

> 1/2  tsp. apple cider vinegar
> 1/2 tsp. honey
> 1 c. water
>
> Optional: add a pinch of cayenne pepper

For a great pick up, mix the above well, and sip with or between meals. (You may need to warm the water slightly in order to dissolve the honey.)
Note: A stock of apple cider vinegar and honey mixture can be made up and kept in the refrigerator. Use 1 tsp. stock per glass of water.

### POTATO PEELING BROTH

> 1 organic potato
> 1 large carrot
> 2 celery stalks
> 1 handful parsley
> 3 c. water

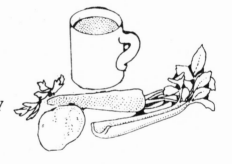

Peel the potato, cutting the peeling 1/4 inch thick. Save the peels. Use the potato in another recipe.
Chop the carrot and celery.
On the lowest possible heat, simmer the potato peels, parsley, chopped carrot and celery for 20 minutes. Strain the vegetables out and save the liquid broth.

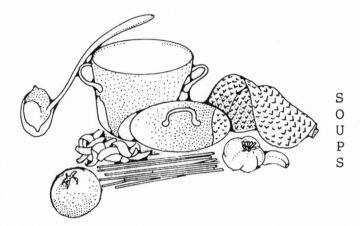

SOUPS

******** S O U P S ********

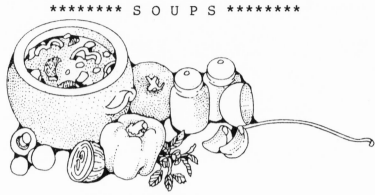

Soups are a wonderful pleasure food. They can be comforting and nourishing on a rainy or cold winter day, or lightly filling when it is too hot to eat. They can be a great appetizer, or a hearty meal in itself.

Soups can also provide creative ways to use left-overs and to add a lot of variety to your diet.

Soups are also perfect for convalescing, and, depending on how they are prepared and which ingredients are used, can provide crucial nourishment for special health problems.

Following are suggested ingredients for soups, suggested techniques for soup preparation, and actual soup recipes.

## SUGGESTED SOUP INGREDIENTS

LIQUID STOCKS:
    water
    water from steaming vegetables
    herb tea
    vegetables juices, warm or cold; fresh
        or pure bottled
    fruit juices, fresh or pure unsweetened
        bottled
    nut or grain milks (see "Beverages")
    vegetable bouillon (water + a bouillon
        cube or powder)
    miso bouillon (see "Miso Soup" recipe)

## SOUP BASES:

Vegetables: fresh, raw vegetables, but
   also left over salad.
   Lightly cooked vegetables and left-
   over cooked vegetables.
   This also includes leafy greens.
Fruits: fresh, or soaked dried
Whole grains: ground or whole, freshly
   cooked or left over.
Beans: freshly cooked or left over
Chicken: freshly cooked or left over
Fish: raw, or freshly cooked
Whole grain noodles: freshly cooked or
   left over
Nuts and/or seeds: whole or ground
Sprouts


## FLAVORINGS:

spices, garlic, leeks, scallions, onions
fresh ginger
olive, sunflower or sesame oil
tahini or almond butter
honey, molasses, maple syrup, barley
   malt or rice bran syrup
apple cider vinegar
soy sauce, miso , kelp or dulse
lemon or lime juice


## THICKENERS:

rolled oats
ground nuts or seeds
ground raw or cooked grain
whole grain flour
kuzu or agar,agar

## SOUP PREPARATION

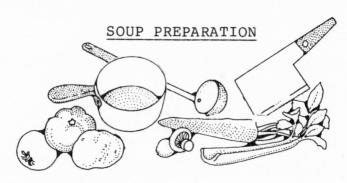

### SOUP COOKED IN A POT:

Prepare as follows:

(a) OPTIONAL: Slightly heat in a soup pot, a small amount of olive oil, butter or water. Add onions or garlic and sauté.

(b) Add any of the following bases:
cooked grain
cooked noodles
cooked fish or chicken
cooked beans
nuts or seeds: ground or whole
lightly steamed vegetables
raw, sliced or chopped vegetables
(If you are going to blend the soup, the vegetables do not have to be chopped very small.)

(c) Add water or stock, covering the soup base. If you want a more liquid soup, add extra stock.

(d) Bring the water or stock close to the boil. Shut the heat off, cover the pot and let the ingredients sit till warm or slightly soft. Root vegetables such as potatoes, turnips, etc. take longer. Don't overcook.

(e) Add spices to taste.

## BLENDED SOUPS

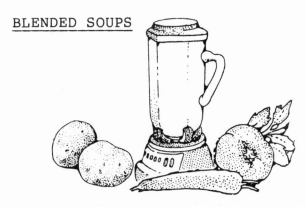

There are many kinds of blended soups. Here are a few varieties with which to experiment:

RAW VEGETABLE #1:

    (a) Slightly chop the raw vegetables.
    (b) Put the vegetables in the blender.
    (c) Add hot or cold stock, as desired, and blend.

For example, see "Quick Gaspacho for One", p.187, and "Quick Borscht", p.186.

Optional:
    Put some of the chopped vegetables aside and add them after blending the other vegetables, if you want a crunchy texture.
    If you want a "creamy" texture, add any of the thickeners listed on page 173, and blend again.

RAW VEGETABLE #2:

    (a) Juice some vegetables
    (b) Add chopped vegetables and spices
    (c) Eat cold, or warm the soup slightly over a low heat
    (d) Blend, or eat as is.

## QUICK CREAMY ROOT VEGETABLE SOUP

(a) Put any vegetables you like in a pot. See "Suggested Combinations" below.

(b) Add enough water, vegetable juice or stock to cover the vegetables.

(c) Bring the water close to the boil, shut the heat off, cover the pot and let the vegetables cook in their own steam.

(d) When the vegetables are slightly soft, put the entire pot contents (liquid plus vegetables) in the blender, and blend.

(e) Add more liquid and/or spices if necessary.

Note: If you want a crunchier texture, don't blend all the vegetables. Put some aside, and add them after blending.

SUGGESTED COMBINATIONS FOR QUICK-COOKED BLENDED VEGETABLE SOUPS:

| | | |
|---|---|---|
| potato | + | garlic and/or watercress |
| potato | + | leek |
| potato | + | celery and watercress |
| potato | + | zucchini and leek |
| carrot | + | leek and dill |
| carrot | + | onion and coriander |
| parsnip | + | scallion and mushroom |
| parsnip | + | butter and/or soy sauce |
| turnip | + | butter and/or soy sauce |
| squash | + | butter and/or soy sauce |
| red potato | + | leek and coriander |
| sweet potato | + | butter and cinnamon |

(Note: Use small amounts of watercress, as it is heavily cleansing, though nutritionally a wonderful food.)

Potato soups are good hot or cold. If you like, add plain yogurt, chopped chives, and/or cucumber. Blend again and refrigerate.

For examples of Blended Cooked Vegetable soups, see pp.186 and 188.

## QUICK CREAMY GRAIN OR BEAN SOUP

The technique described on the previous page can be used to prepare a creamy grain or bean soup, but the grains or beans will have to be cooked more than the vegetables. For example, for quick, creamy split pea or lentil soup, low-simmer 1/3 c. split peas or lentils and two cups water for 40 minutes. Then blend the beans and the water. Refer to the grain and bean cooking charts, pp.251 and 271 for cooking times.
Three good combinations of creamy bean soup are the following:
> Cooked barley + water + parsley
> Cooked aduki beans or black beans + water + small amount chopped celery leaves + small amount grated lemon peel


## BLENDED LEFT OVERS:

(a) Put left over salad, steamed vegetables, cooked grains or beans in the blender.
(b) Add hot or cold water, soy or nut milk, or stock.
(c) Blend and add spices to taste.

For example: Zucchini-tomato sauté (see vegetable sauté, p.226.) is delicious blended with fresh or pure bottled tomato or vegetable juice. It makes a quick Gaspacho soup.

Another example: Blend cooked pumpkin, squash, carrots or sweet potato with your favorite soy milk or nut milk and/or water. For extra flavor, add sautéed scallions and a little butter. Herbs can also be added to taste, such as dill added to the carrot soup.

## CREATE-A-SOUP

Another excellent technique for preparing soups is by using your steamer to create your own soup recipe. Simply steam some ingredients over a broth for about 10 minutes. Then add the steamed ingredients to the broth.

The broth can be water or juice, such as tomato or beet juice. You can also create a miso broth by adding miso paste. Add it after cooking; otherwise, you will destroy the beneficial properties in the miso and alter the flavor.

Herbs or spices, such as garlic or ginger can be added to the broth before the steaming begins. As the broth simmers under the steamer, the herbs will add flavor to the broth and to the ingredients being steamed.

While the broth is simmering, other foods can be cooked in the broth underneath the steamer, such as fish or noodles. This works well if you are preparing a quick soup for one person, since you won't need a large amount of fish or noodles. Larger amounts won't fit underneath the average steamer.

Ingredients to put in the steamer are any of the following: Vegetables, fish, cooked chicken, cooked grain or cooked beans.

It takes only about 8-10 minutes to cook the vegetables, fish or noodles, or to warm the cooked chicken, grain or beans.

After the ingredients in the steamer are cooked or warmed, empty them into the broth. If you prefer a "meal" to a soup, you can separate the ingredients out from the broth. See Create-A-Meal, p.227.

On the following page is a chart showing 6 different types of soups which you can create with this technique. Use these as examples to stimulate your own creativity. The advantage in this technique is that it is fast, and you can use foods on hand.

## CREATE - A - SOUP

These delicious, hearty soups take minutes to prepare; Use the same format to create your own recipes.

| SOUP | BROTH LIQUID | BROTH INGREDIENTS | INGREDIENTS TO STEAM | ADDITIONAL INGREDIENTS |
|---|---|---|---|---|
| MISO | 1 c. water | - | 1/2 c. diced tofu<br>1/3 c. sliced Jerusalem artichoke | 2 tsp. miso stirred with the broth until dissolved.<br>1 Tbl. chopped scallions. |
| VEGETABLE | 1/4 c. water<br>3/4 c. tomato juice | 1 tsp. thyme | 1 small carrot, sliced<br>1 small carrot, sliced<br>1 small potato, diced<br>1 ripe tomato, chopped<br>1/4 zucchini, sliced | 1 Tbl. chopped parsley<br>Cayenne pepper to taste |
| CHICKEN NOODLE | 2 c. water | 1 large clove garlic, minced<br>1 oz. whole grain fettucini noodles | 6 okra, sliced, after removing the ends (or, use 1 stalk celery, chopped)<br>1 c. chopped, cooked chicken (without skin)<br>2 Tbl. sliced mushrooms | 1 Tbl. chopped parsley<br>1/2 tsp. tarragon |
| TOMATO FISH | 2 c. water | 1 large clove garlic, minced<br>1 tsp. thyme | 1 tomato, chopped<br>3/4 c. diced, raw fish (such as cod or haddock) | 1 Tbl. chopped parsley<br>Cayenne pepper to taste |
| MISO FISH | 2 c. water | 1 large clove garlic, minced<br>2 tsp. minced ginger | 1 small carrot, sliced<br>3/4 c. diced, raw fish<br>3 1"pieces wakame seaweed | 2 tsp. miso, stirred into the broth until dissolved |
| BEET | 1/2 c. water<br>1/2 c. beet juice | 1 tsp. caraway seeds | 1/4 c. sliced leeks<br>1/2 c. chopped cabbage | Optional: 1 Tbl. kefir cheese or plain yogurt |

DIRECTIONS:
Put the broth liquids in a medium sized pot ( 8 1/2" x 7" is perfect). Bring the liquid close to a boil. Add the "Broth Ingredients". Turn the heat down to a low simmer. Put a vegetable steamer in the pot. Put the "Ingredients to Steam" in the steamer. Cover the pot. Simmer on a low heat for 8 minutes, or until the vegetables are slightly soft, and the chicken is warm, or the fish is cooked. Turn the heat off. Empty the steamed ingredients into the broth. Add the "Additional Ingredients". Serves 1.

******** SOUP RECIPES ********

(Also see Soup Preparation Techniques, pp.174 through 179.)

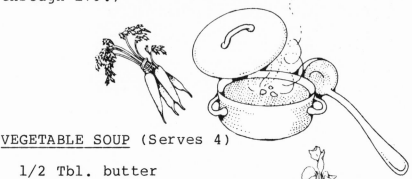

VEGETABLE SOUP (Serves 4)

1/2 Tbl. butter
1 large onion, chopped
1-2 cloves garlic, minced
4 c. water
1 vegie cube or 1 tsp. powder
2 carrots, chopped
1 leaf cabbage, torn into pieces
2 stalks celery, chopped
1 potato, diced
1/2 turnip, diced
2 tomatoes, diced
1 small bay leaf
1/8 tsp. thyme

Melt the butter on a low heat in a large pot. Add the onions and garlic and sauté till soft. Add the water. Stir the vegie cube or powder till dissolved. Add the remaining ingredients.
Bring the water close to the boil. Turn the heat off, cover the pot and let the vegetables sit till slightly soft, but still crunchy.

Optional:
        Add cayenne pepper to taste, after cooking.
        Add miso paste as per instructions under "Miso Soup", p.182.

## QUICK CHICKEN OR FISH NOODLE SOUP
(Makes about 2 1/2 c.)

    1 clove garlic, minced
    4 large mushrooms, chopped
    1 tsp. butter
    2 c. water
    1 oz. whole grain noodles
    1/4 tsp. thyme
    1/2 c. sliced okra (optional)
    1 c. diced cooked chicken or diced raw
      fish (such as cod or haddock)
    1 Tbl. chopped parsley
    1/2 large tomato, chopped
    pinch cayenne pepper

Melt the butter on a low heat on a soup pan.
Add the garlic and mushrooms. Sauté till they
are soft. Add the water, noodles and thyme.
Low simmer 5 minutes. Add the remaining
ingredients, except the cayenne, and low
simmer another 3 minutes. Add the cayenne.


## ONION SOUP (Serves 4)

olive oil          1 minced clove garlic
6 medium sized white onions, sliced thin
pinch cumin        1/2 tsp. mustard
6 c. water         1 vegie cube or 3 tsp. powder

Cover the bottom of the pot with a thin layer
of olive oil. Heat the oil slightly, then add
the onions, garlic, and mustard. Sauté on a
low heat till the onions are lightly brown.
Add a pinch of cumin, the water and the vegie
cube.
Bring the water just to the boil, cover the
pot, then turn the heat down to a low simmer
for about 45 minutes.
Before serving, add 2 tsp. soy sauce, and
more cumin and cayenne pepper to taste.

## MISO SOUP (Serves 4)

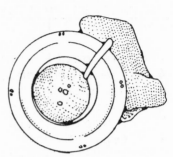

4 c. water
A few pieces of seaweed
    (wakame or dulse)
4 scallions, chopped
3 carrots, sliced or
    diced
4 Tbl. miso paste

Optional:
   1/2 cube of Tofu, broken into small chunks
   1 Jerusalem artichoke (sunchoke), sliced
   Minced garlic, and/or ginger to taste

Put the seaweed, scallions and carrots in the water in the pot.
(Add the minced garlic and/or ginger and the sunchokes at this point.)
Bring the water close to the boiling point. Add the tofu, cover the pot, turn the heat off, and let the vegetables sit, covered, till slightly soft (8 to 10 minutes).
Put the miso paste in a cup or small bowl. Ladle a small amount of the soup broth into the bowl and stir till the miso is dissolved. Empty the miso broth into the soup and stir. Do not let miso boil, as it stops the beneficial enzyme activity, and distorts the flavor.

Note: Miso broth makes a great, hearty soup base, especially for a winter soup.

For a quick miso soup for one person, see "Create-A-Soup", p.179.

LENTIL-TOMATO SOUP (Serves 6)

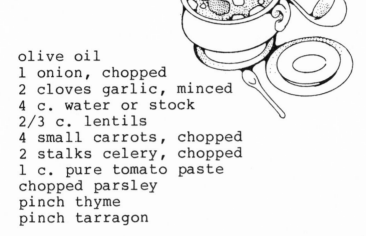

olive oil
1 onion, chopped
2 cloves garlic, minced
4 c. water or stock
2/3 c. lentils
4 small carrots, chopped
2 stalks celery, chopped
1 c. pure tomato paste
chopped parsley
pinch thyme
pinch tarragon

Optional:
  Add cayenne pepper and/or freshly grated parmesan cheese after cooking, to taste.

Sauté the onion and garlic on a low heat in an oiled soup pot.
Add the water and lentils.
Bring the water close to the boil, then turn the heat down to the lowest possible setting. Cook for 45 to 60 minutes, or until the lentils are soft.
When the lentils are soft, add the carrots and celery. Cover the pot and turn the heat off. Let sit, covered, till the vegetables are slightly soft (8 to 10 minutes).
Stir in the tomato paste, then add the spices to taste.

ALTERNATES:
        Omit the tomato paste.
                    and/or
        Use barley in place of lentils.

LEMON-EGG SOUP (Serves 2-3)

(This is a great way to use left over rice)

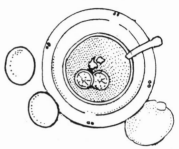

3 c. water
3 bouillon cubes
4 large cloves garlic
1 bay leaf
1 cup cooked brown rice
1 Tbl. butter
2 eggs
juice of one lemon

for garnish: one thin slice of lemon per serving

Bring the water to a boil in a soup pot. Add the bouillon cubes, the bay leaf and the garlic. Simmer at the lowest possible temperature for 30-40 minutes, allowing the garlic flavor to permeate the water.
Remove and discard the bay leaf and garlic.

A few minutes before the above process is completed, heat the rice in a separate pan in the butter, and beat the eggs in the lemon juice.

About 5-10 minutes before serving the soup, add some of the hot broth mixture to the beaten egg/lemon mixture. Stir vigorously, then return the broth/lemon/egg mixture to the soup pot.

Continue to stir the soup broth and to heat it for a few minutes on a low temperature, until the egg mixture is smoothly blended into the broth.

Add the cooked rice and serve at once.

Garnish each bowl of soup with a paper thin slice of lemon, and, if you like, a sprig of parsley or watercress.

---

## BLENDED SOUP RECIPES

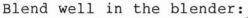

### RAW SPINACH SOUP
(Makes 3 cups)

Blend well in the blender:
  1/4 c. almonds
  1 c. tomato juice
  1 c. water
  2 c. raw spinach
  1 small clove garlic, minced
  1 Tbl. chopped scallion (1 thin scallion)
  1/2 c. packed celery leaves
  3/8 tsp. ground cumin (or) 1/8 tsp. ground
    nutmeg
  1/8 tsp. kelp, dulse powder or vegetable
    salt

After blending the above mixture, gradually add and blend in a second cup of water, blending to the consistency you like.

Note that the taste will be completely different if you use nutmeg in place of cumin. If you aren't sure which to use, empty small amounts of the mixture into two cups. Then add a pinch of nutmeg to one cup, and two pinches of cumin to the other. They are both good!

## RAW BORSCHT (Makes 4 cups)

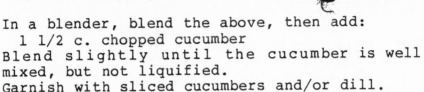

```
3/4 c. fresh or pure bottled beet juice
1 1/2 tsp. dried dill, or caraway seeds
1/2 tsp. soy sauce
1 Tbl. lemon juice
1 clove garlic, minced
1 1/4 c. water
1/3 c. tomato juice
```

In a blender, blend the above, then add:
  1 1/2 c. chopped cucumber
Blend slightly until the cucumber is well mixed, but not liquified.
Garnish with sliced cucumbers and/or dill.


  For a QUICK COLD BORSCHT for one person, blend 1 small beet, 1 c. water, chopped cucumber (3 times more cucumber than beet), and lemon juice, dill or caraway to taste.
  For a delicious hot borscht for one, which does not require a blender, see Create-A-Soup p.179.

PLEASE NOTE: For some people, beet juice will stain their eliminations red.
  Beets, though a great liver support, are heavily cleansing, so do not use more than a beet the size of a golf ball per person, or 1/3 c. juice per person.


## SWEET POTATO OR SQUASH SOUP (Makes 6 cups)

In a blender, blend well:
  4 c. cooked sweet potato or winter squash,
    such as pumpkin, acorn or butternut
  2 1/2 c. water
  2 Tbl. melted butter
  1/3 c. chopped scallion, lightly sauteed
    in butter

GASPACHO (RAW VEGETABLE)
(Serves 4)

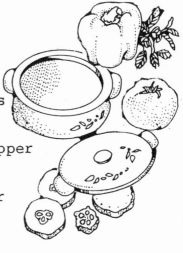

    1/2 c. water
    2 c. tomato juice
    2 tsp. lemon juice
    3 Tbl. chopped scallions
        (about 1 scallion)
    1 clove garlic, minced
    2 Tbl. chopped green pepper
    1 tsp. basil
    1/2 tsp. chervil
    2 pinches cayenne pepper
    1/2 tsp. kelp
    1 Tbl. chopped parsley
    1 small cube of a beet

Blend the above thoroughly in the blender,
then add:

    1 c. chopped tomatoes
    1/2 c. chopped celery
    1/2 c. chopped zucchini
    2 c. peeled and chopped cucumber
        (about 1/2 cucumber)

Garnish with parsley and a slice of lemon.


QUICK GASPACHO FOR ONE

    Blend any fresh vegetables (or left
over, such as the tomato-zucchini sauté - see
p.226.) in one cup fresh or pure-bottled
tomato juice.

---

## POTATO LEEK SOUP
(Serves 4)

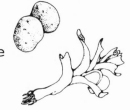

   3 Tbl. butter
   3 large potatoes, sliced fine
   2 medium sized leeks, sliced
   1 1/2 c. water
   1/2 tsp. mustard
   1 c. plain yogurt
   parsley to garnish

Melt the butter on a low heat in a large saucepan. Add the potatoes, leeks, mustard and water. Bring the water close to the boiling point. Shut the heat off and let sit, covered, till the potatoes and leeks are slightly soft.
Blend the entire pot contents in the blender, adding more water if you like. Add the yogurt and blend again. If necessary, rewarm, but be careful not to boil, as it spoils the yogurt and gives it a metallic taste.


## QUICK POTATO SOUP FOR ONE

   1 1/2 c. water
   1/2 large potato, chopped in chunks

Put the potato and the water in a soup pot. Bring the water close to the boil. Cover the pot, shut off the heat and let the potato cook in its own steam till slightly soft.
Put the potato and water in the blender and blend well.
If you like, add any of the following while blending:

   butter    soy sauce    chives    cucumber
   minced garlic    watercress    parsley

USE THIS SAME FORMAT FOR ANY ROOT VEGETABLE: PARSNIPS, TURNIPS, DAIKON RADISH, CARROTS, ETC.

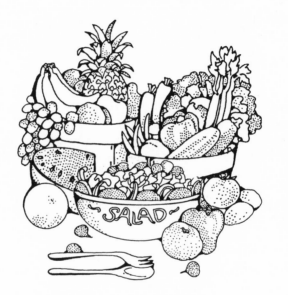

S
A
L
A
D
S

******** S A L A D S ********

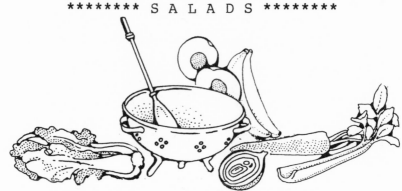

Salads can be the most important part of your meal, since they can provide you with a variety of nutrients, fiber and vitality. And, they can give you the most pleasure - in their beauty, their delicious taste, and in their opportunity for you to be creative.

Salads can be created from any type of food in any combination. Experiment with the varieties of colors, flavors, textures and shapes. This is Mother Nature's way of letting us know we are getting a good variety of nutrients, without needing to know the chemical breakdown of foods.

Experiment to your heart's delight.


## SUGGESTED SALAD INGREDIENTS

Cooked grains            Cooked beans
Cooked noodles           Tofu
Cooked chicken           Sprouts
Cooked or raw fish
Vegetables: chopped, sliced, grated,
    diced, or eaten finger-sized.
Leafy greens such as romaine lettuce,
    parsley, watercress, raw spinach, etc.
Fruits: fresh, or dried and rehydrated
    (soaked).
Nuts and seeds: whole, ground, soaked or
    chopped.
Fresh herbs or flowers

****** VEGETABLE & FRUIT SALAD RECIPES ******

Please note: For noodle salads, grain salads, bean salads and chicken salads, refer to the individual sections.

If you are not sure of the identification of certain vegetables, such as Jerusalem artichoke (or sunchoke), see the drawings on pages 44-45.

## QUICK SALADS

### SALAD ON THE GO

Washing and chopping ahead of time is generally not recommended, since it results in loss of nutrients and vitality. Occasionally, however, you could pre-cut and refrigerate some leafy greens and raw vegetables. Eat them as a quick snack with a dip. Or, combine them in a last-minute salad and mix with a pre-made dressing.

You could also pre-cook beans, grains and chicken. Keep them in separate containers. Combine them as you like with the vegetables and/or cooked noodles. Again, top with a pre-made dip or dressing, such as the tofu dip, p.205, mustard dressing, p.275, or Ruth Duffy's Tarragon Dressing, p.202.

### CARROT SALAD

    4 c. grated carrots (about
       3 medium sized carrots)
    1/2 c. chopped walnuts
    1/2 c. soaked currants or raisins
    1 c. diced apples and/or pineapple
    2 Tbl. shredded coconut
    Optional: add 1/2 c. sunflower seeds

Mix and decorate with sprigs of parsley
Top with "honey dressing", p.204.

## AVOCADO-WATERCRESS

Combine sliced avocado and
watercress leaves. (Save the
hard watercress stems for your
green drink.)
Squeeze lemon juice over the
avocado and watercress, then
sprinkle soy sauce on top.

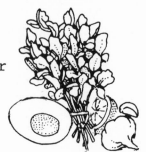

Optional additions:
sesame seeds       tofu chunks        raw peas
raw zucchini       raw string beans   sprouts
slices of raw Jerusalem artichoke (sunchoke)

NOTE: For a longer (but delicious!) version
of the avocado watercress salad, and to serve
4 people, use 3/4 bunch of watercress leaves
and 1 ripe avocado. Top with the following
sauce:
    4 Tbl. raw green olive oil
    2 cloves garlic, minced
    4 tsp. sesame seeds
    2 Tbl. soy sauce
    2 1/2 Tbl. lemon juice

Sauté the garlic in the oil, on a low heat,
for approximately 2 minutes, stirring constantly. Add the sesame seeds. Continue to
sauté for 1 minute longer, taking care that
the seeds don't burn. Remove from heat. Add
the soy sauce and lemon juice. Make a bed of
watercress on 4 individual salad plates. Top
with sliced avocado, then the dressing.

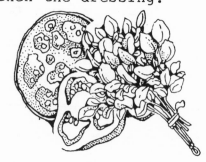

## TOMATO-BASIL

Slice a fresh, ripe
tomato. Top with
fresh basil and a
good quality olive
oil.

## BLENDED SALAD

In a blender, blend well in the order listed:
    Juice from 1/2 lemon
    1 Tbl. sesame or sunflower oil
    1 wedge of a ripe tomato
    1 small cucumber, sliced
    1/2 green pepper
    2-3 leaves romaine lettuce
    1-2 stalks celery
Optional: Add spices of your choice, such as minced garlic or a pinch of cayenne pepper.

This salad will have a "mush" texture. It is an excellent "salad" for those who have extreme dental or digestive difficulty.

## WATERCRESS-ENDIVE SALAD

    1 c. sliced endive
    1 c. watercress sprigs (Save the hard stems for your green drink.)
    12 pecans, chopped

Mix, and top with "Ruth Duffy's Tarragon Dressing", p.202. This salad is delicious with "Italian Tofu Noodles", p.265.

## AVOCADO-SUNCHOKE SALAD

    3 Jerusalem artichokes (sunchokes - see picture, p.44.), sliced thin
    1 ripe avocado, pitted, peeled and diced
    1/2 c. mung bean sprouts
    1/4 c. alfalfa sprouts
    1 c. shredded Romaine lettuce

Mix all ingredients well, then sprinkle with lemon juice to taste.

## RAW VEGETABLE SNACKS

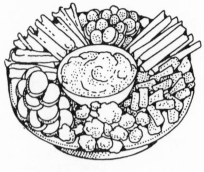

Raw vegetables are
wonderful snacks -
plain, or with dips
or sauces. Use any
of the following:

| | |
|---|---|
| cherry tomatoes | raw peas |
| carrot slices | celery slices |
| broccoli flowers | green string beans |
| turnip slices | radish roses |
| sweet potato slices | yellow snap beans |
| sliced bell peppers | mushroom bulbs |
| cauliflowerettes | cucumber slices |
| sliced Jerusalem artichokes (sunchokes) | |

Arrange the vegetables in a beautiful manner
in baskets or on a plate. Put the vegetables
on a bed of romaine and/or purple head
lettuce and decorate with slivers of purple
cabbage, radish roses, cherry tomatoes and
large sprigs of parsley or watercress.

Or, carry them in a baggie as a snack, along
with a container of nut butter or dip. (See
"Dip" recipes, p.205.)

## PEA SALAD (Serves 3)

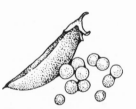

1 c. fresh raw peas
1/2 c. grated red cabbage
1/2 c. sliced sunchokes
2 Tbl. chopped scallions
1/4 c. chopped green beans
2 Tbl. sliced radish
2 Romaine or Boston lettuce leaves, torn
   into bite sized pieces.

Combine, and top with tofu dressing, p.205.

## ALFALFA CROQUETTES (Serves 2)

Mix thoroughly:
    1 c. alfalfa sprouts
    2 Tbl. grated red cabbage
    2 Tbl. grated carrot
    4 Tbl. chopped celery
    2 Tbl. chopped parsley
    1/2 tsp. minced garlic
    2 Tbl. tahini
    1 tsp. lemon juice
    3 Tbl. carrot juice
    1/2 c. ground sunflower seeds (about 1/3 c.
       unground seeds)

Serving suggestions:
(1) Serve in tomato cups. Cut the tomato
    about 3/4 of the way down, 3 ways, so that
    you have 6 sections connected at the
    bottom. After you fill them with the
    mixture, top with parsley sprigs and serve
    on a bed of lettuce.
                    (or)
(2) Refrigerate the mixture for 1 hour, so
    that it is more stiff, then form patties.

## MARINATED VEGETABLES

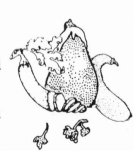

    1/4 eggplant, peeled and diced
    3/4 lb. yellow squash, diced
    3/4 lb. zucchini, sliced thin
    1 small red onion, sliced thin
    1/4 c. chopped parsley

Marinade:
    1/4 c. olive oil                 1/4 tsp. basil
    1/4 c. apple cider vinegar       pinch oregano
    1 small clove garlic, minced

Marinate the vegetables for 5 hours or more,
stirring occasionally. Decorate with parsley.

## SALT FREE
## SAUERKRAUT

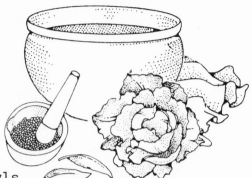

UTENSILS:
    3 mixing bowls
    a large crock ware or glass pot
    a plate which fits just inside the pot
    a clean, white cotton cloth
    a heavy weight, such as a water-filled jar

INGREDIENTS:
    1 head green cabbage and 1 head purple
        cabbage, grated, except for the outer
        leaves. Put the outer leaves aside.
    2 onions, chopped
    8 cloves garlic, minced
    2 carrots, grated
    2 zucchini, chopped
    1 head cauliflower, broken into flowerettes
    2 stalks celery, chopped
    2 beets, grated
    2 Tbl. each of caraway seeds, dill seeds
        and celery seeds. Measure, then grind.
    1 Tbl. ground kelp
    2 Tbl. garlic powder

This recipe may look slightly complicated, but doing it is very simple and very rewarding. It is delicious and will keep refrigerated for weeks. Sauerkraut is an excellent source of vitamins C, B1, B2, thiamin, and riboflavin, as well as calcium, phosphorous, and lactic acid, which helps maintain a healthy bowel. The sauerkraut ferments in 8 to 10 days. It also makes great sauerkraut juice in the process.
This recipe makes several quarts. Small quantities can be prepared in the same way.

-196-

SAUERKRAUT PREPARATION:

Put the grated cabbage in one mixing bowl, the prepared vegetables and onion in another bowl, and the ground spices and minced garlic in another bowl.

Put a layer of the cabbage about 1" deep in the crock ware or glass pot. Pack it down. Put a 1" layer of the vegetable mixture over the cabbage and pack it down. Then sprinkle with a layer of the spices. Gently mix the entire mixture and pack it down again.

Repeat the process until you are finished with the ingredients, or until you are 3" from the top of the pot. (You need space, since the water you will add will bubble and rise in the fermentation process.)

Cover the mixture with the outer leaves of the cabbage, tucking the leaves around the mixture as well as possible. Cover the leaves with the cotton cloth and tuck the cloth tightly around the mixture.

Pour water (or rejuvelac, if you want it to ferment faster. See recipe under "Beverages".) over the cloth and keep pouring until you see that the sauerkraut is well drenched and water is appearing above the cloth.

Put the plate on top, then the weight. Push the plate down to be sure the mixture is packed as tightly as possible.

Put a clean cloth over the pot, and put the pot in a warm place (about 70-80° F). If it has not started bubbling within 48 hours, the place is not warm enough. You can put the pot in the oven with the pilot light.

Be sure there is always enough liquid above the plate, since the liquid keeps the sauerkraut from spoiling.

When it is ready (8-10 days), skim off the fuzz, or skum, on the surface. Gently remove the weight, plate, cloth and outer leaves plus any more fuzz. Drain and mix the sauerkraut, saving the juice, then refrigerate the juice and sauerkraut.

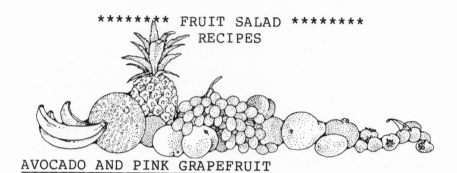

******** FRUIT SALAD ********
RECIPES

## AVOCADO AND PINK GRAPEFRUIT

Pit, peel and slice a ripe avocado. Cut out the sections of the grapefruit. Arrange the pieces on a bed of lettuce and top with poppy seed dressing , (p.204) and a sprig of watercress.
Optional: Add chopped pecans.


## TROPICAL DELIGHT

Combine in a bowl:
| | |
|---|---|
| sliced bananas | green grapes |
| sliced or diced papaya | soaked currants |
| (or) | |
| sliced or diced mango | strawberries |
| diced pineapple | |

Optional: add shredded coconut.

Eat as is, or top with thick almond milk, or Quick Fruit Dressing, p.201.

Please note: An easy and less messy way to prepare a mango is as follows:
Cut just through the skin (not into the fruit) of the mango, all the way around, from end to end, on two sides. Hold the mango and peel one section, exposing the fruit. With a knife, cut the fruit off the pit. Keep peeling and cutting fruit, holding an unpeeled section as long as possible. Eventually, there will be no more unpeeled section to hold, but this method helps get more fruit off the pit with less mess.

D
R
E
S
S
I
N
G
S

D
I
P
S

&

S
A
U
C
E
S

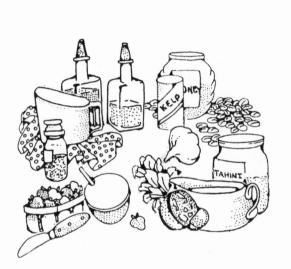

```
******** D R E S S I N G S ********
      D I P S  &  S A U C E S
```

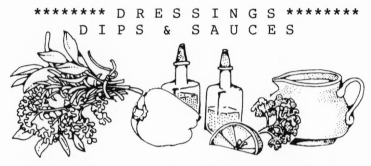

SAUCE, DIP AND DRESSING INGREDIENTS :

Oils

    Cold pressed olive, sesame, sunflower,
        walnut, flax or soy
    Nut/seed butters, such as tahini, almond
    Avocado

Liquids

    Water
    Vegetable juices
    Fruit juices or concentrates
    Apple cider vinegar

Bulk Ingredients

    Vegetables: raw, lightly steamed
    Fruits: fresh or rehydrated dried
    Cooked beans
    Cooked grains
    Tofu
    Ground nuts and seeds

Flavorings

    Fresh & dried herbs and spices
    Sweeteners such as honey, molasses,
        maple syrup, barley malt, fruit juice
    Soy sauce
    Lemon or lime juice

Thickeners

    Flour
    Kuzu or Arrowroot (See pp.207 and 208.)
    Slippery elm powder or ground psillium
        seeds)

-200-

******** SALAD DRESSING RECIPES ********

Salad dressings can be made
by mixing oil, vinegar or other
liquids with herbs and spices.
Or, in a blender, blend any
fruits and vegetables with
liquid ingredients and
seasonings.
Many of the dressing recipes can be used for
sauces, and some of the dip recipes can be
used as dressings simply by adding more
liquid for a thinner consistency. Each recipe
will note this possibility.


## SUPER QUICK DRESSINGS

LEMON/SOY: Squeeze lemon juice over
steamed or raw vegetables, or avocado. Then
sprinkle soy sauce on top.

OIL/VINEGAR: Sprinkle apple cider
vinegar or lemon juice over the salad, then
add the oil and spices.

GINGER/SOY: Mix minced ginger, soy
sauce and lemon juice, then put on the salad.

QUICK CARROT: Blend tofu, carrot, soy
sauce and lemon juice to taste.

BLENDED VEGETABLE: In a blender, blend
any vegetables (such as tomato, green pepper,
or lettuce) with apple cider vinegar, olive
oil, herbs and minced garlic.

QUICK FRUIT DRESSING OR SAUCE: In a
blender, blend any fruits, by themselves or
together, with a small amount of water or
pineapple juice. Optional: Add to taste
honey, vanilla or cinnamon.
Suggested fruits: peach, pineapple, banana.

## OIL AND VINEGAR

    2-3 Tbl. apple cider vinegar
    1 pinch cayenne pepper
    1 tsp. dried basil
    1 clove garlic, minced

Combine the above, then add:
    1/4 c. sesame oil
    1/4 c. olive oil

Variations, add any of the following:
    a pinch of powdered kelp
    1/3 tsp. soy sauce
    1-2 sprigs parsley, finely chopped
    pinch grated parmesan cheese

## SUNFLOWER/BEET DRESSING

    1/2 c. sunflower seeds
    1 c. beet juice, fresh
        or pure bottled
    1 1/2 tsp. soy sauce
    1 1/2 tsp. lemon juice
    1-2 cloves garlic, minced
    1/4 c. each of sesame and olive oil
    1 1/2 tsp. dill, or to taste

Grind the sunflower seeds in a dry blender.
Add the beet juice, soy sauce, lemon juice
and garlic. Blend. Then, while the blender is
on low, slowly add a steady stream of the 1/2
c. mixture of olive and sesame oil. Add dill.

## RUTH DUFFY'S TARRAGON DRESSING

Blend well in a blender:
1 c. sesame oil          1/3 c. cider vinegar
1 Tbl. tarragon          1 tsp. celery seed
3 cloves garlic, minced  1 tsp. mustard

## TAHINI-GINGER DRESSING OR SAUCE

    1" piece of ginger, peeled and minced
    3 garlic cloves, minced
    1 c. oil (half sesame, half olive, for ex.)
    juice of 1 lemon
    2 Tbl. each tahini and soy sauce

Place the garlic and the ginger in a blender.
Cover with a little oil and blend to a fine
paste. Add the rest of the oil, lemon juice,
tahini and soy sauce. Blend again. Add more
tahini if a thicker dressing is desired.

This is also a delicious sauce for grains,
noodles or tofu.

## WATERCRESS DRESSING

Combine in a blender and blend well:
    1/2 c. mayonnaise
    1 c. plain yogurt
    1 c. chopped watercress leaves
    1 Tbl. apple cider vinegar
    1 Tbl. fresh lemon juice
    1/2 tsp. soy sauce
    1/2 tsp. minced onion
    1 clove garlic, minced

## CARROT-GINGER DRESSING

3 Tbl. sesame seeds
1 medium carrot, cut in 1 " pieces
1/2 c. olive oil          4 tsp. soy sauce
2 Tbl. cider vinegar      1/2-3/4 c. water
1 1/2 - 2 tsp. minced  fresh ginger

Grind the sesame seeds and set aside. Chop
the carrot pieces in your blender, then add
sesame seeds and other ingredients and blend.

## SWEET DRESSINGS

Also See Super Quick Fruit Dressing, p.201.


HONEY DRESSING (Makes 1/3 cup)

Combine and shake well before using:
   1/2 c. sunflower or sesame oil
   2 Tbl. honey
   1/4 tsp. lemon juice


BANANA DRESSING (Makes 1 cup)

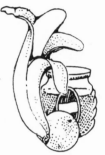

Blend well in a blender:
   1/2 c. sunflower or sesame oil
   1/2 c. pineapple juice
   1 Tbl. lemon juice
   1 medium sized, ripe banana


POPPY SEED DRESSING (Makes 1 cup)

Blend well in a blender:
1/3 c. honey              2 tsp. onion juice
1/4 tsp. dry mustard   2 tsp. poppy seeds
1/2 c. sesame or sunflower oil
1/4 c. apple cider vinegar
1 tsp. lemon juice
1/4 tsp. grated lemon peel


PAPAYA DRESSING (Makes 1 1/2 cup)

Mix well:
   1/2 c. sunflower or sesame oil
   1/2 c. papaya concentrate
   1/2 c. apple cider vinegar
   1 Tbl. lemon juice

Optional: If a mayonnaise is preferred, whip
an egg into the mixture.

******** DIP RECIPES ********

To make these dips into dressings or sauces, simply add more liquid.

For a quick dip, use nut butter, such as tahini or almond butter. Add chopped cucumber for a lighter taste.

For other dip ideas, see p. 207.


## TOFU-VEGETABLE DIP, SAUCE OR DRESSING

3/4 c. light olive oil
1 medium sized carrot, slightly chopped
2/3 c. chopped fresh parsley
1 tsp. white part of scallion
1 Tbl. green part of scallion
3 Tbl. lemon juice
1 clove garlic, minced
8 oz. firm tofu
1 Tbl. soy sauce

Put the olive oil and the carrot chunks in a blender and blend well. Add the parsley, scallions, lemon juice and garlic and blend well. Then add the tofu and soy sauce. Blend well again. It comes out thick, like a dip. For a sauce over steamed vegetables, or for a salad dressing, add water to thin.

Note: For a curried tofu dip, see p. 260.


## GUACAMOLE (AVOCADO DIP)   Serves 4

2 ripe avocados, pitted and mashed
1/8 tsp. onion juice
1 1/2 Tbl. lemon juice
12 ripe cherry tomatoes, chopped
1 large, or two small scallions, chopped

Mix all ingredients well, adding the avocado last. Serve in a bowl as a dip or spread.Or, serve in the avocado skin or in tomato cups.

## SESAME TAHINI DIP, SAUCE OR DRESSING

    1/4 to 1/2 c. lemon juice
    1 scallion, chopped
    2 cloves garlic, minced
    1/2 green pepper, seeded and chopped
    1/4 c. chopped parsley
    1/2 c. water
    1 c. tahini
    1 pinch cayenne pepper
    1/2 tsp. cumin
    2 Tbl. soy sauce

Put the garlic, lemon juice, scallion, green pepper and parsley into the blender. Blend well until smooth.
Add the water. Then, while the blender is on low, slowly add the tahini. If it's still too thick, add more water.
Add the remaining spices and blend again.

This recipe makes a blender full of a great dip for raw vegetables. For a dressing or sauce for vegetables, grains, noodles, tofu, or beans, add more water until the consistency desired.

## SPRING GREEN DIP (Makes about 1 1/2 c.)

    2 Tbl. finely chopped of each: red pepper
        and green pepper
    3 Tbl. finely chopped of each: parsley and
        scallions
    2/3 c. plain yogurt
    1/2 c. mayonnaise
    pinch cayenne

Mix the mayonnaise and the yogurt in a bowl, then add the vegetables.
Add the cayenne.
Mix well and chill.
Serve with mixed raw vegetables.

******** SPREADS & SAUCES ********
RECIPES

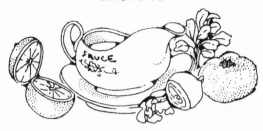

Put sauces on cooked grains, noodles, tofu, legumes (beans), chicken or fish, loaves or steamed or raw vegetables.

Use the same ingredients as suggested for soups (see p.172), only use less liquid for a thicker consistency.

## THICKENERS

For thickening sauces, see p.200 for a list of thickeners. Two particularly good thickeners and jelling agents (which are wheat free) are kuzu and arrowroot. See "Glossary" for information on these starches.

### Kuzu

There are many advantages to using kuzu as a thickener or gelling agent:

(1) It has a smooth, light texture and a delicate, non-starchy flavor.

(2) By adding it to sauces or frostings, you extend the amount of sauce without adding caloric ingredients such as tahini or honey, or salty ingredients such as miso.

(3) When used in sweet sauces or glazes, the alkalizing properties of the kuzu help balance the acidic properties of the sweet.

To use kuzu, mix it with cool liquid, blending or stirring till dissolved. Crush any lumps with your fingertips. If necessary, strain. Otherwise, put the mixture over a very low heat and stir constantly till thick.

The proportions of kuzu and liquid are:
Sauces: 1 1/2 to 2 1/4 tsp. kuzu to 1 c.
liquid, depending on the thickness of
the sauce.
Jells: 2 Tbl. kuzu to 1 c. liquid

## Arrowroot

Arrowroot is less expensive than kuzu,
but lacks kuzu's alkalizing and medicinal
properties and is inferior in texture. It
does not make as smooth and delicate a sauce,
nor as firm and cohesive a jell. However, it
is perfectly adequate.

Use 1 1/2 Tbl. arrowroot per cup of
liquid to be thickened. Mix it with a small
amount of the liquid first. Stir until it has
dissolved and is the consistency of paste,
then add it to the simmering liquid, which
will then turn cloudy. Continue stirring
until the liquid is clear and thick. Remove
from the heat and let cool.

## QUICK SAUCE OR SPREAD COMBINATIONS:

Blend well in any proportions preferred. Add
water to thin, if necessary:

Mix by hand in a bowl:
* Miso paste or soy sauce + tahini and any
  flavorings (See recipe, p.209.)
* Tahini + ginger
* Tahini + dulse seaweed and lemon juice
* Tahini + honey or barley malt + cinnamon
  (great on toast)
Blend in blender:
* Cooked millet + tahini and soy sauce
* Cooked rice + tahini and ginger
* Cooked potatoes + butter, garlic and soy
  sauce
* Cooked lentils + garlic, lemon juice and
  soy sauce
* Tofu + tahini, ginger and soy sauce

## QUICK BLENDED SUPER SAUCE OR GRAVY

Put in the blender:

| | |
|---|---|
| 1 1/2 c. water | 1 Tbl. kuzu |
| 1/4 c. tahini | 1 Tbl. miso |
| 2 tsp. minced ginger | |

Blend well, then cook on a low heat, stirring constantly, till thick. Refrigerate, covered.

### Alternates:

Make the above gravy; however, eliminate the ginger and add any of the following:

    1 clove garlic, minced.
    1 1/2 tsp. ground cumin (or) 1 tsp.
     tarragon


## MISO-TAHINI SPREAD OR SAUCE

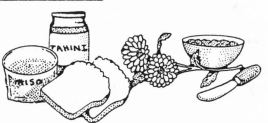

1 c. tahini
1/4 - 1/3 c.
  miso paste
water to thin

Add the miso to the tahini gradually, to taste, as miso is very salty. Add water, stirring very well, to thin. ( A small amount of water, such as 2 Tbl., will still give you a spread, yet will soften the flavor and extend the amount.) Refrigerate, covered

Use any of the following optional flavor changers:

| | |
|---|---|
| 1-2 tsp. honey | lemon juice |
| grated fresh ginger | 1/2 tsp. marjoram |
| 1 Tbl. minced onion or garlic | |
| grated orange or lemon peel (organic) | |

As a spread, it's delicious on bread, toast or crackers with sprouts or chopped watercress leaves. Or, use it as a sauce.

## TOMATO SAUCES

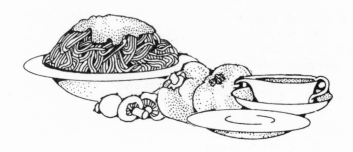

**REAL TOMATO SAUCE** (Makes about 2 1/2 c.)

    1/4 c. olive oil
    1 very large onion, diced
    3-4 cloves garlic, minced
    1/4 c. chopped mushrooms
    1/4 green pepper, chopped
    2 Tbl. diced parsley
    1 tsp. oregano
    2 tsp. basil
    1 bay leaf
    3 1/2 c. skinned and chopped tomatoes. (If
you cannot find large, ripe tomatoes, use
ripe unpeeled cherry tomatoes, or two 12 oz.
cans unadulterated canned tomatoes.)


Sauté the onion, garlic and mushrooms in the
olive oil till the onions are lightly
browned. Add all other ingredients. Bring
close to the boil, then reduce heat to lowest
possible simmer. Simmer 45 minutes. Add
water if it gets too thick.

---

## NO-TOMATO TOMATO SAUCE (makes about 4 cups)

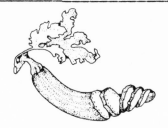

(For those allergic to tomatoes, here is a sauce that tastes very much like tomato sauce.)

      2 Tbl. olive oil
      1 1/2  large onion, chopped
      3 cloves garlic, minced
      1 Tbl. chopped parsley
      1/2 green pepper, seeded and chopped

Sauté the onion and garlic in the olive oil till the onion is well transparent. Put aside 1/2 c. of the onion/garlic mixture, the parsley, and 1 Tbl. of the chopped green pepper.
In a blender, blend well the following:

    The remaining sautéed onion/garlic mixture
    The rest of the green pepper
    2 medium sized zucchinis, chopped
    1 small to medium sized beet, chopped
    2 Tbl. Italian seasoning (Such as, 1 1/2
        Tbl. basil, 1 tsp. oregano and 1 tsp.
        thyme)
    2 tsp. apple cider vinegar
    1 Tbl. minced garlic
    1 1/2 Tbl. olive oil
    2/3 c. water (or more, if necessary)

After blending, return the blended mixture, along with the ingredients you put aside, (1/2 c. onion/garlic mixture, 1 Tbl. chopped green pepper and 1 Tbl. chopped parsley) to the pan and let gently simmer on a low heat until the flavors are well blended. You may want to add more apple cider vinegar, olive oil or water.

******** JAMS & RELISHES ********

## STRAWBERRY JAM

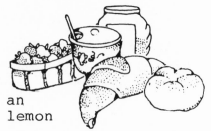

Blend well:
    2 c. strawberries
    1/2 c. honey
    1 section each of an
       orange and of a lemon

(You may occasionally need to turn off the
blender and use a rubber spatula to push the
ingredients into the center of the blender.)

ALTERNATES: Use dried apricots, which have
been soaked for 2-3 hours. Or, use fresh
peaches and eliminate the orange and lemon.


## GINGERED CARROT MARMALADE

    1 c. grated carrots          2 Tbl. water
    3/4 unpeeled organic lemon, sliced (remove
       seeds)
    1 1/2 to 2 tsp. minced ginger.
    1/2 c. honey
    1 Tbl. pure pectin (no sugar or chemicals)

Put the carrots, lemon, ginger and water into
a blender. Blend to a coarse mixture. Put the
mixture in a bowl. Add the honey and pectin.
Mix well. Refrigerate 3 hours, or overnight.
NOTE: If you don't like ginger, just
eliminate it for a delicious honey marmalade.


## CRANBERRY RELISH (Makes 1 1/2 c.)

    2 c. cranberries             1/2 c. honey
    1 small organic orange, with peel,
       cut in pieces.

Grind the cranberries in the blender, then
add the orange pieces and the honey.

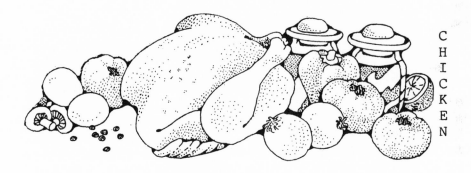

C
H
I
C
K
E
N

******** C H I C K E N ********

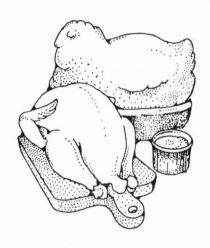

    Chicken has about the same nutritional value as red meat, yet is less expensive, has less fat, and is easier to digest. However, commercial chickens are fed arsenic to stimulate appetite, and are injected with antibiotics and hormones to encourage quick, fatty growth and fast profits. Whenever possible, buy organically raised chickens. The extra cost will be balanced by increased health value.

    The following chicken recipes are delicious, but sometimes it's easier and more creative to have chicken pre-baked in the refrigerator to add to salads, soups, or other recipes at the last minute. See "Create-A-Soup", p.179, "Create-A-Meal", p. 227, and Bean Salad, p.275, for recipe ideas.

******** CHICKEN RECIPES ********

COQ AU VIN
(Serves 4-6)

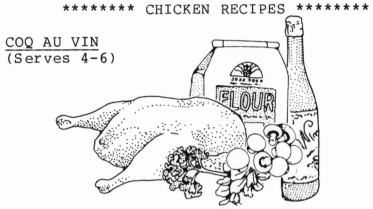

Use a broiler or roasting chicken or 2
   fryer chickens, cut into parts.
4 Tbl. whole wheat or rye flour
4 Tbl. corn meal
3 Tbl. butter
3/4 c. diced onions
1 clove garlic, minced
6 shallots or small white onions
8 large, whole mushrooms
1 medium carrot, sliced
2 Tbl. chopped parsley
1 small bay leaf
1 Tbl. chervil or marjoram
1/4 tsp. thyme
1 1/2 c. dry red wine or sherry

Preheat the oven to 325°. Wash the chicken
pieces and pat them dry.
Mix the flour and cornmeal and roll the
chicken pieces in it till the pieces are well
covered.
Melt the butter in a large fry pan. Brown the
chicken in the butter, then put the chicken
in a large casserole which has a lid.
Sauté the diced onions and garlic in the
juices in the fry pan.
Add the sautéed onions and garlic, the juices
from the fry pan and all remaining ingredients to the chicken in the casserole. Cover
and bake until done - about 1 1/2 - 2 hours.

CURRIED CHICKEN
(Serves 2)

    1 small fryer chicken, quartered
    2 Tbl. whole grain flour
    2 Tbl. cornmeal
    1/4 c. butter
    1 onion, chopped (about 1 1/2 c.)
    1 clove garlic, minced
    5 mushrooms, chopped (about 1 1/3 c.)
    2 Tbl. curry powder
    2 Tbl. cumin
    1/2 Tbl. turmeric
    1/4 Tbl. cardamon
    2 whole cloves
    1 Tbl. plain yogurt
    1/2 c. tomato juice

Wash the chicken, pat dry and dip into a mixture of the flour and cornmeal. Brown the chicken in butter in a large fry pan or stove-top casserole.
Remove the chicken and put it aside to drain and let cool to touch.
Gently simmer in the casserole the onion, garlic, mushrooms and spices. (Add more butter, if you need it.)
Debone and skin the chicken and cut it into bite sized pieces.
Add the chicken to the pan. Stir it into the spices until the pieces are coated. Add the yogurt, tomato juice and enough water until there is a sauce (about 1 c.). Simmer gently about 1/2 hour. Add more spices, water or tomato juice, if necessary.

NOTE: For a quick-cook curried chicken, use 4 baked boneless chicken breasts. Skin them and cut them into bite sized pieces. Sauté the onion, garlic, mushrooms and spices in 3 Tbl. butter. Add the chicken, yogurt and tomato juice. Simmer till flavors blend (about 1/2 hour).

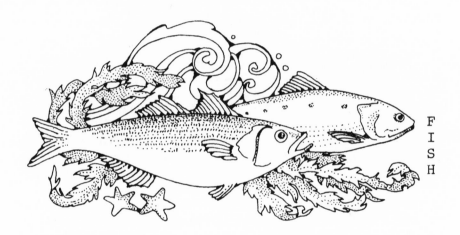

F
I
S
H

******** F I S H ********

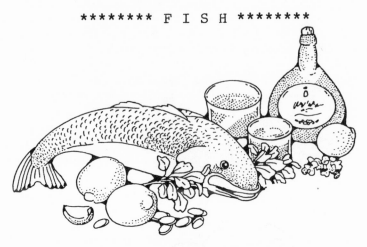

Fish meat is very delicate, and therefore deteriorates rapidly. It is difficult to
be sure of freshness by its appearance, since
freezing methods mask the age, but in
general, the eyes bulge and are bright, with
a black pupil and transparent cornea; the
gills are reddish pink; the scales adhere to
the skin and have a sheen to them; the odor
of the fish is non-offensive, especially
around the gills or belly, but smells something like seaweed. The flesh of the fish is
firm to the touch and bounces back when you
touch it, rather than forming an imprint.
Fresh fish, when placed in cold water, will
float rather than sink. The real criterion
for freshness, however, is how it keeps after
you buy it, its odor and appearance when you
prepare it and, finally, of course, its
taste.
      Eat shell fish in moderation, as they
are very rich and difficult to digest, and,
since they are by nature scavengers, may be
contaminated. Also avoid, if possible,
shallow water fish since they are more likely
than deep ocean fish to be exposed to environ-
mental pollutants, such as pesticides,
chemical waste, laundry detergents, etc.,
that are carried from land to water.[1]

Choose inland fish from lakes which you know are pure, - far from "civilization". Or choose deep ocean fish, especially the smaller variety, such as mackerel, herring, sardine, or flounder, which are lower on the food chain and therefore less likely to be polluted. Other deep ocean fish are bass, bluefish, butterfish, cod, haddock, halibut, red snapper, sea bass, sea trout, shad, the soles, swordfish, tuna, turbot and whiting.

Fish should be cooked quickly, since after a certain point (150°) the delicate tissues break down and the nutritious juices are lost. Broiling should never take longer than 10 minutes, and baking, at 375°, should take a maximum of 1/2 hour for a whole fish. Fish is generally "done" <u>before</u> the point at which it flakes easily with a fork.

For other recipes using fish, see "Create-A-Soup", p.179, and "Create-A-Meal", p.227.

******** FISH RECIPES ********

<u>QUICK FISH FOR ONE</u>

    1/4 lb. filet of
        flounder or sole
    2 Tbl. water
    2 Tbl. soy sauce
    1 inch ginger, minced

Put the fish in a low pyrex baking dish. Add enough water and soy sauce and ginger to just barely cover the fish. Put the dish into the broiler and broil approximately 5 minutes. While broiling, spoon some of the liquid mixture over the fish.

Optional: Marinade the fish in the mixture for 1/2 hour before broiling.

## BROILED FISH IN LEMON SAUCE (Serves 4)

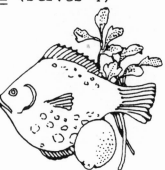

1 lb. fish fillets such
    as scrod or sole
Sauce:
  1/3 c. melted butter
  1 clove garlic, minced
  1 Tbl. lemon juice
  1 Tbl. chopped parsley.

Note that other herbs, such as dill or tarragon in place of, or with parsley, are also delicious. Use tarragon on chicken.

Wash the fish and pat dry. Put it into a pan which will fit in the broiler. Lightly saute the garlic in the butter. Let cool slightly, then add the lemon juice and parsley. Brush both sides of the fish with the sauce, and broil 4-5 minutes on one side only.

## FISH ORIENTALE (Serves 4)

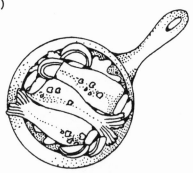

1 lb. fish fillets,
    such as flounder,
    sole, or scrod.
3-4 Tbl. butter
4 slices fresh ginger
3 Tbl. water
1/4 c. soy sauce
2 scallions, chopped

Heat the butter in a large fry pan. Add the fish, and cook till it is lightly brown on both sides. Drain most of the butter, then add soy sauce, scallions, water and ginger. Cover and simmer 5 minutes. Turn the fish and simmer another 5 minutes till done. Add a pinch of cayenne pepper, if you wish.

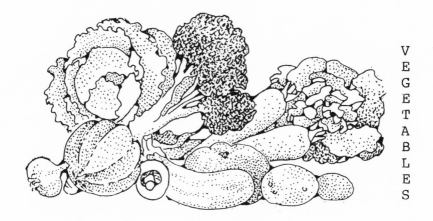

V
E
G
E
T
A
B
L
E
S

******** V E G E T A B L E S *********
ENTRÉES AND SIDE DISHES

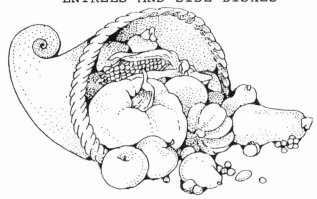

To get the most out of your vegetables, eat them raw or very lightly cooked. Boiling vegetables destroys 20-45% of the minerals, 75% of the natural sugars, a large percentage of the vitamins, and all of the enzymes and life force. Enzyme destruction begins at 130°.

Over cooking vegetables also renders their fiber useless as bulk. Raw vegetables are the very best form of fiber. See "Salads" and "Soups" for raw vegetable recipes.

COOKING VEGETABLES

Vegetables, if cooked, should be steamed, baked, or gently sautéed on a low heat in a little olive oil or butter.

Vegetables can also be made into wonderful soups. See "Soups".

Please note that vegetables containing oxalic acid should be eaten raw, or barely heated. High heat converts the organic oxalic acid into an inorganic substance which inhibits calcium assimilation and may result in the formation of crystals of calcium oxalate in the kidneys. Vegetables in this category are rhubarb, mustard greens, Swiss chard, kale, collards, French sorrel, spinach, asparagus and beet greens.

Vegetables are "done" when they are slightly soft, but still have a crunchy texture and good color.

Most people find that rather than using specific recipes for cooking vegetables, they prefer to steam or sauté vegetables, or eat them raw, in various combinations that come to mind at the time of preparation, with ingredients that are easily available. Pages 226 and 227 contain information and a technique, "Create-A-Meal", that I hope will help stimulate your own creativity.

## STEAMED VEGETABLES

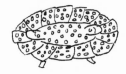

Vegetables can be steamed together, or by themselves on a stainless steel, ceramic or bamboo steamer.

To steam most vegetables, bring the liquid under the steamer close to the boil, shut the heat off, cover the pot and let the vegetables cook in their own steam. It takes only minutes. This works especially well for the softer vegetables, although root vegetables will cook this way as well.

To steam especially hard vegetables, such as artichokes, bring the liquid under the steamer close to the boil, then turn it down to the lowest possible simmer, and let the vegetables cook, covered, till done.

Steaming vegetables over a broth instead of plain water adds a hint of flavor. Use miso broth, vegetable broth, soy sauce and water, or garlic and water.

Use spring or distilled water for steam water, then save it for a soup base, for a broth, or add it to sauces.

## SAUTÉED VEGETABLES

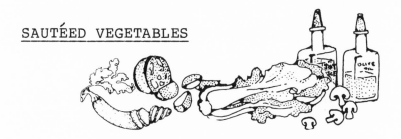

(Note: "Sauté" means lightly stirring on a low heat in a small amount of butter or olive oil. No frying, please!)

Plan on about 2 1/2 c. cut raw vegetables per serving. Cut in bite sized, thin slices to cook quickly and retain crispness.

Before sautéeing vegetables, separate them into three groups:
(1) onions and/or garlic

(2) harder, longer cooking vegetables, such as carrots, potatoes, green string beans, cauliflower

(3) softer, quick cookers such as zucchini, mushrooms, peppers, tomatoes

Put the vegetables in group (1) in the pan first, as they take the longest, then add those in group (2), then those in group (3).

One delicious, quick example is tomato-zucchini sauté. Sauté minced garlic, sliced zucchini and chopped tomatoes in olive oil till slightly soft. Add basil and/or grated parmesan cheese.

## ADD TO SAUTÉED OR STEAMED VEGETABLES:

butter        soy sauce        lemon juice
butter and soy sauce
butter and lemon juice
tofu or tahini sauce (see Sauce recipes)
ground nuts and seeds
sprouts
chopped parsley
minced garlic
cooked grain, noodles and/or beans
grated parmesan cheese

## CREATE-A-MEAL

The chart on the following page uses a fast and easy technique for creating whole meals using vegetables and any other foods, such as chicken, fish, whole grains, noodles or beans.

Simply steam your choice of ingredients over a broth in which other ingredients are cooking at the same time. When all ingredients are cooked (about 8 to 10 minutes), remove them from the steamer and from the steaming water. The ingredients can then be combined together or eaten separately. For example, if you cook noodles under the steamer and cook vegetables at the same time in the steamer, after they are cooked you can add the vegetables to the noodles, or eat them separately.

Top the cooked ingredients with a little butter, soy sauce, miso/tahini sauce, or any other sauce of your choice.

This technique works especially well when cooking for one person, since small amounts fit well under the steamer.

Use these 6 different meal examples to stimulate your own ideas. Also see p.179, "Create-A-Soup", for other ideas for ingredients.

## CREATE - A - MEAL in a pot

These are quick, easy, delicious meals which serve 1. To make more, double the ingredients. Use this format to create your own recipes.

| MEAL | POT INGREDIENTS | STEAMER INGREDIENTS | OPTIONAL SAUCE |
|---|---|---|---|
| SPICEY SOBA NOODLE | 1 oz. buckwheat soba noodles<br>2 c. water | 1 small carrot, sliced<br>2 tsp. minced ginger<br>1/2 c. chopped tofu<br>3 Tbl. sliced mushrooms<br>1/2 c. snow peas<br>2 Tbl. chopped almonds | Miso-tahini sauce with cayenne pepper added to taste |
| SUNCHOKE NOODLE | 1 oz. whole grain fettucini noodles<br>2 c. water | 1 c. diced cooked chicken<br>1/2 c. chopped sunchokes (Jerusalem artichokes)<br>1/2 c. fresh green peas<br>1/4 c. sliced mushrooms | Miso-tahini sauce with tarragon added to taste (Use less miso than usual) |
| POACHED FISH | 4 oz. fish fillet<br>2 c. water | 1 c. chopped broccoli<br>1/2 c. sliced leeks | lemon juice, minced garlic and parsley |
| VEGETABLE SPAGHETTI | 1 oz. whole grain spaghetti noodles<br>2 c. water | 1 c. sliced zucchini<br>1 c. chopped tomatoes<br>1/4 c. chopped parsley | Tomato sauce and grated parmesan cheese |
| GINGER FISH & VEGIES | 1 oz. whole grain noodles<br>2 tsp. minced ginger<br>2 c. water | 3/4 c. diced raw fish (ex:haddock,cod)<br>1 small carrot, sliced<br>1/2 c. chopped broccoli<br>1/2 c. chopped cauliflower | Quick blended Super Sauce over the noodles, or over the combined ingredients |
| FISH 'N RICE | 4 oz. fish fillet<br>2 c. water | 1 c. cooked wild rice<br>3 Tbl. chopped almonds<br>1/4 c. sliced leeks<br>2 Tbl. chopped parsley | Sprinkle with soy sauce |

DIRECTIONS:
Put the 2 c. water in a pot. Bring it close to a boil. Add the other "Pot Ingredients".
Turn the heat down to a low simmer. Put a vegetable steamer in the pot. Put the "Steamer Ingredients" into the steamer. Cover the pot.
Simmer on a low heat for 8 minutes. After 8 minutes, or when the vegetables are slightly soft, gently remove the steamer with the "steamer ingredients".
Strain the water off the "Pot Ingredients" - that is, off the noodles or fish.
You may now either combine the steamer ingredients with the pot ingredients (the noodles or fish), or eat them separately.
Use the "Optional Sauce" over the combined or separated ingredients.

RECIPES FOR VEGETABLE
ENTRÉES AND SIDE DISHES

## QUICK VEGETABLE CASSEROLE

Steamed or baked vegetables can be mixed or blended with an egg, melted butter and any spices, and, if you like, cooked grain. Then, lightly butter a casserole dish, put the mixture in the dish and bake. For example, add cooked broccoli to the rice-cheese nut loaf, p.253.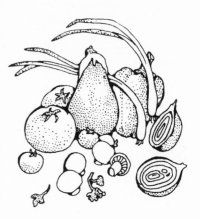

Or, put the pre-cooked mixture in a pre-made pie crust for a vegetable pie. See "Sweet Potato Scallion Pie", p.235, for an example.

## VEGETABLE FOO YUNG (Serves 4)

       2 Tbl. sesame oil
       1 onion, finely chopped
       1 clove garlic, minced
       2 Tbl. sesame seeds
       2 c. shredded Chinese cabbage
       1 c. snow peas
       1  8 to 10 oz. cake tofu, in chunks
       1/2 c. sliced water chestnuts
       1/4 c. soaked Chinese mushrooms

Slightly heat the oil in a fry pan. Add the garlic, onion and sesame seeds and sauté till the onion is transparent. Add all ingredients but the sprouts and stir till slightly soft. Add sprouts and soy sauce to taste.

## FLOUR-FREE VEGETABLE PIE

3 large potatoes, sliced thin
   (no more than 1/4" thick)
5 Tbl. butter
1 clove garlic, minced
2 medium zucchini, sliced thin
1/4 tsp. each: basil and oregano
2 ripe tomatoes, sliced thin
a mixture of 1/2 c. grated swiss cheese
and 1/2 c. grated parmesan or goat cheese

Preheat the oven to 400°.
Melt the butter in a pan. Add the garlic.
Dip the potato slices in the garlic butter.
Line the bottom and sides of a 9" pie plate
with one layer of potato. Put one layer of
zucchini on top of the potato, layering to
the edge of the plate. Sprinkle the herbs on
top of the zucchini. Add a layer of tomato,
then the cheese.
Bake at 400° until the potatoes are crispy
and the cheese is browned (about 1 hour).


## ALL-AMERICAN PIZZA

Use a whole grain English muffin*
   Amounts per muffin half
   one slice of tomato
   1/8 tsp. minced garlic
   pinch dried oregano and basil
   1/4 tsp. olive oil
   1 Tbl. grated hard cheese
   1/8 tsp. grated parmesan

Lightly toast the muffin. Top with a slice
of tomato, the garlic and spices, then the
oil and cheese. Bake at 350° until the
cheese is melted and the tomato soft.

*NOTE: For a large pizza, use a large whole
grain biale or pita bread.

## SUNBURGERS

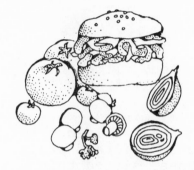

There are many varieties of nut burgers. Experiment on your own, using different kinds of vegetables and nuts and seeds.

Sunburgers can be eaten raw, as well as cooked. Just use less onion and garlic.

Top sunburgers with tomato sauce or sugar-free ketchup, called "table sauce", since it cannot be called ketchup unless it contains sugar.

In a pinch, sunburgers freeze well.

## SUGGESTED INGREDIENTS FOR SUNBURGERS:

(These ingredients make about 6 burgers:)

    1 1/2 c. freshly ground sunflower seeds
        (about 1 c. unground seeds)
    2 Tbl. chopped onions (small pieces)
    1 clove garlic, minced
    1/2 c. grated carrots (about 1 medium sized
        carrot)
    1/2 c. small pieces chopped celery (about
        1 large stalk)
    2 Tbl. chopped parsley
    2 tsp. chopped green pepper
    2 Tbl. wheat germ (omit if allergic to
        wheat)
    1/8 tsp. basil
    1/2 tsp. soy sauce
    1 egg, beaten
    1 Tbl. sesame or olive oil
    1/4 c. tomato juice, or water

## SUNBURGER PREPARATION

Mix sunflower seed meal, vegetables and spices, except the soy sauce.

In a separate bowl, mix the beaten egg, oil and soy sauce, then add that to the vegetable mixture.

Thoroughly combine the two mixtures, then add juice or water to make a doughy consistency.

Shape into patties and arrange on an oiled baking sheet.

At 350° bake 15 minutes on one side, then turn the patties and bake 10 minutes more.


## BLENDED SUNBURGERS

If you have a strong blender, the ingredients for the sunburger can be chopped and mixed in the blender.
Grind the seeds, put them aside, then add the carrots, celery and green pepper (which have been chopped slightly) and the rest of the ingredients. Blend well, then add to the sunflower meal.

## BROCCOLI QUICHE

(This is great "transition food" for those who think "health food" can't taste good)

### QUICHE CRUST (Makes one 9" crust)

    3/4 c. whole wheat flour
    1/4 c. wheat germ
    1/2 c. (1 stick or 8 Tbl.) butter
    2 Tbl. ice water
Optional: 1/4 tsp. sea salt

Put a small glass of water in the freezer so that the water will be icey cold when it is time to measure the 2 Tbl. of water.
Put a stick of butter out on the counter so it is slightly soft when needed.
Preheat the oven to 425°.
Mix the flour, wheat germ (and salt) in a large bowl.
Cut the butter into the flour with a pastry blender until the mixture looks like pea-sized crumbles. Sprinkle the water into the flour mixture and stir lightly with a fork. Handle as little as possible.
Flour a piece of wax paper and the rolling pin. Roll out a 10 1/2" circle of the flour mixture onto the wax paper.
Gently uncurl the wax paper from the dough circle, placing the dough in the pie pan.
The dough edges should be slightly thicker, particularly if you wish to flute them.
Prick the bottom of the crust in several places with a fork.
Bake the crust at 425° for 8-10 minutes, or until it just begins to turn lightly brown.

-232-

If you wish to make 2 pie shells, and freeze one for next time, use these proportions:

1 1/2 c. whole wheat flour    2/3 c. butter
1/2 c. wheat germ            1/4 c. ice water

## BROCCOLI QUICHE FILLING

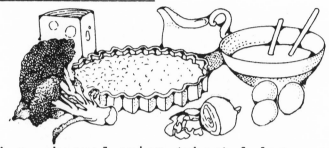

1 3/4 c. chopped onion (about 1 large
    onion)
1 c. grated gruyere or Swiss cheese
1/4 c. grated parmesan cheese
3 eggs, beaten
2 c. (1 pint) heavy cream
1/8-1/4 tsp. nutmeg
2 1/2 c. chopped broccoli (1 bunch). Use
   flowerettes and thin slices of the stem.

Preheat oven to 425°.
Slightly steam the broccoli.
Sauté the onion in butter till slightly clear (a couple of minutes), then put the onion in the bottom of the baked crust.
Mix together the grated Swiss and parmesan cheese, then put the mixture in the crust.
Add the broccoli.
In a separate bowl, beat the eggs, then add the cream and nutmeg.
Pour the egg/cream mixture into the crust, covering the vegetables and cheese evenly.
(You probably won't need the whole egg/cream mixture.)
Bake for 15 min. at 425°, then reduce heat and bake at 350° for 30-40 minutes more, or until the top is lightly brown.

## RAW FERMENTED SEED LOAF

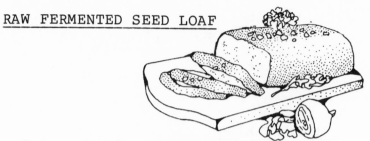

3 c. ground sesame seeds
3 c. ground sunflower seeds
1 c. ground almonds
1 green pepper, chopped
1 onion, chopped
2 stalks celery, chopped
3 cloves garlic, minced
1 c. parsley, chopped
1 Tbl. basil and 1 tsp. thyme
1/2 tsp. each oregano and marjoram
     pinch cumin
Optional: 1 tsp. powdered kelp, and/or,
       1 to 2 Tbl. soy sauce

Mix the ingredients in a large bowl. Add enough water or rejuvelac (fermented grain water - see p.167) to make a dough. You will need only about 2 to 3 Tbl. liquid, since the loaf becomes much more moist as it ferments. It is better to use rejuvelac, since the enzymes in the rejuvelac help digest the heavy protein of the nuts and seeds.
Leave the loaf in a warmish place, or at room temperature for 24 to 28 hours. Cover it with a damp cloth to keep it from drying out. The longer it sits, the more fermented it will become, and the tangier the taste.
Serving Suggestion: Slice a green pepper, remove the seeds and put a small amount of seed loaf inside. Top with a slice of tomato and a sprig of parsley. Or, spread the loaf on crackers with parsley, tomato and sprouts.

PLEASE NOTE: Eat SMALL amounts. No more than 1/2 c. at a time. It's very concentrated.

## SWEET POTATO SCALLION PIE

Crust:
    3/4 c. brown rice flour
    1/2 c. oat flour
    1/3 c. butter, slightly soft
    3 Tbl. ice water

Preheat the oven to 400°.
Lightly oil a 9" pie pan.
Combine the flours in a large bowl. With a
pastry blender, cut the butter into the flour
till you have pea sized crumbles. Sprinkle in
the ice water, mixing briefly with a fork.
Form the mixture into a ball.
Lightly flour a piece of wax paper larger
than 11" round. Also flour a rolling pin.
Roll out a circle of the mixture, about 1/4"
thick and 10 1/2" round, onto the wax paper.
Gently unroll the wax paper from the dough
circle, placing the dough in the pie pan.
Flute the edges, if you wish.
Prick the bottom of the crust in several
places with a fork.
Bake at 400° for 10 to 12 minutes, or until it
just begins to turn lightly brown.

Filling:
    2 Tbl. melted butter
    1/4 c. chopped scallions
    1 egg
    2 c. cooked sweet potato (2 large sweet
        potatoes - approximately 1 1/4 lb.)
    1/2 c. soy or nut milk, or water
    1/2 c. water

Melt the butter in a small fry pan. Lightly
saute the scallions in the butter.
Beat the egg in a large bowl, or blender. Add
the cooked sweet potatoes, milk, water and
butter/scallion mixture. Beat with an electric beater, or blend in a strong blender
till smooth. Pour the filling into the crust
and bake at 400° for 45 minutes to 1 hour.

## BAKED SQUASH WITH WILD RICE STUFFING

(Use acorn or butternut squash.)

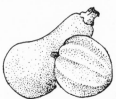

Slice the squash in half from end to end. Remove the seeds. Turn the squash face down on a lightly oiled pan. (This keeps it from drying out.) Bake at 350° for 45 minutes. Meanwhile, prepare the stuffing.

### Stuffing
    3 Tbl. butter
    1 clove garlic, minced
    1 Tbl. chopped onion
    2/3 c. chopped mushrooms
    2/3 c. whole grain bread cubes
    3 tsp. dried parsley
    1 tsp. dried thyme
    3/4 c. cooked wild rice
    1/3 c. chopped celery

Crush the dried parsley and thyme in a mortar or cup.
Sauté the minced garlic, chopped onions and mushrooms in the butter. Add the bread cubes and crushed herbs. Stir well till combined, then add the rice and celery. Mix.
Makes enough to fill the cavities of both halves of the squash.

After the squash bakes face down for 45 minutes, turn it face up and fill the cavities with the stuffing. Bake another 15 to 20 minutes.

### Alternative to the stuffing
For a sweet alternative to the stuffing, fill the cavities with a pad of butter and 2 Tbl. gingered carrot marmalade (See p.212.)

## SUPER EASY SIDE DISHES

### TOMATOES PROVINCAL (Serves 4)

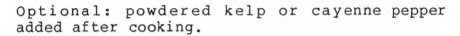

4 ripe tomatoes
2 tsp. basil
1 tsp. oregano
2 cloves garlic, minced
1/4 lb. Swiss cheese, grated,
  or mozzarella, sliced
1 Tbl. grated Parmesan
      cheese
1 1/2 Tbl. olive oil
1/2 tsp. butter

Optional: powdered kelp or cayenne pepper added after cooking.

Slice the tomatoes in half. Put them in a lightly oiled baking dish. Sprinkle the tomatoes with basil and oregano, then with the Swiss and parmesan cheese.
In a small pan, melt the butter on a low heat, then add the olive oil and minced garlic. Sprinkle this mixture over the tomatoes.
Bake at 350° for 45 minutes.

### SWEET POTATO PUDDING

1 cooked sweet potato
1 egg
2 Tbl. butter
Nutmeg, cinnamon and/or allspice to taste.

Blend well in a blender. Add water if this is too thick.

Some people love this for breakfast.

## HERBED POTATO

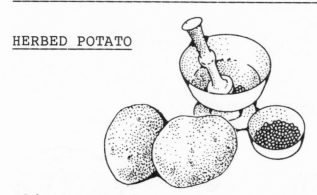

Slice a baking potato in half, leaving the jacket on. Butter it lightly on the cut end. Place it in a pan, cut end down, on a thin bed of caraway or cumin seeds. Bake at 350° till done (about 45 minutes).

## POTATO PANCAKES (Makes 12 pancakes)

1/2 c. chopped onions
2 1/2 c. grated potato (approximately 1 lb. mature potatoes)
2 tsp. soy sauce
2 eggs
2 Tbl. brown rice flour

Sauté the onions in butter, till lightly browned.

Put the grated potato in a clean white cotton cloth or cheese cloth. Thoroughly squeeze out the excess moisture. (You may need to press a small amount of potato at a time. If you use cheese cloth, you can rinse it out afterwards and use it again.)

Beat the eggs in a large bowl. Add the soy sauce, onions and potato. Mix well, then add the flour and mix again.

Form patties of the mixture. Cook them in butter in a fry pan till lightly browned. You will need to turn them.

Serve with plain yogurt, kefir cheese or homemade apple sauce.

## STEAMED ARTICHOKE

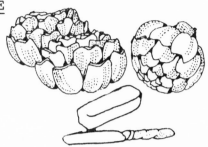

Choose an artichoke that is fairly tight without any brown spots and that "squeeks" when you gently squeeze it. Cut off the stem. Pull off the tough bottom row of leaves and, if you like, cut off the prickly tips with scissors.
Place the artichoke upright on a steamer. Bring the water to the lowest possible simmer, and cover the pot. Steam for about 45 minutes till the leaves pull off easily.
Drain and serve hot or cold.

Artichoke Sauce:
Use a traditional hollandaise sauce, or mix melted butter and lemon juice, and, if you like, minced garlic.

## STEAMED GARLIC BROCCOLI (Serves 1-2)

    3/4 c. broccoli flowerettes
    1/4 c. sliced broccoli stem
    3/4 c. sliced leek (the white part and the
        tender green part)
    1 clove garlic, minced

Steam the broccoli stems. When slightly soft, add the flowerettes, the leek and the minced garlic. Steam till slightly soft.

Suggested Additions:
Melted butter and/or lemon juice and/or soy sauce.

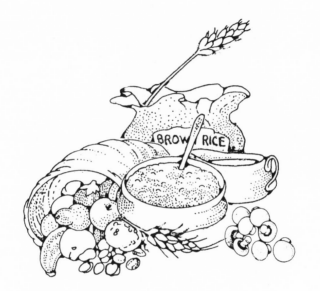

G
R
A
I
N
S

******** G R A I N S ********

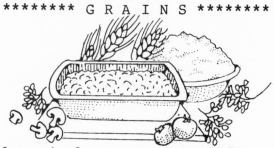

Use only whole, unprocessed, unrefined grains. Refined grains have been stripped of almost all nutrients - Vitamin E, protein, B vitamins and other vitamins and minerals,- as well as fiber, so necessary for good health.

Keep grains (as well as flour, nuts and seeds, and oils) in the refrigerator or freezer to help avoid rancidity and bug infestation.

Grains can be sprouted or cooked ground or whole, eaten as cereals, side dishes, in casseroles, patties, soups, sauces, broths, or in various mixtures with other grains, beans, vegetables and nuts and seeds. (See "Cereals", "Sauces", "Beverages", "Soups" for other grain recipes.)

All grains should be rinsed in cold water before cooking, in order to remove excess starch and grit and to begin the swelling process. Put the grain in a large pot. Add enough tap water to cover. Swirl the grain around. Drain. Repeat if necessary, until the water is clear.

Remember that in soaking or cooking grains, they increase in volume, so use a pot large enough to accomodate the increase. Use a non-aluminum pot with a tightly fitting lid, as the grains should cook in their own steam.

Use approximately 1/4 - 1/2 cup dry grain per person. For a side dish or for breakfast, 1/2 - 3/4 cup cooked grain per person is sufficient, and for a main course, 1 cup cooked grain per person.

Sometimes you will come across a difference in grain hybrids, such as short grain or long grain rice. Short grain will come out tender and moist, and is best for most recipes. Long grain is better in recipes for rice stuffing, or for soups.

Cook grains slowly on as low heat as possible to preserve the most nutritional value and life force. To help you cook on a low heat, use a flame tamer or bent wire in-between the pot and the flame.

To help avoid mushy grains, do not stir them except where indicated. Once the pot lid is on and the grains are cooking, try not to peek until the cooking time is up.

Grains are ready to eat when they are chewy, and not overly soft or too hard. If you want a porridge, blend the cooked grain with a liquid and, if you like, soaked dried fruit, nuts or seeds, soy sauce, tahini, miso, etc. (See "Cereals" recipes.)

The preparation of grains can spark much creativity by combining them with various ingredients listed below. Though it is always best to eat freshly cooked grain, some people find it helps to cut down on their stress load, and helps them avoid less positive foods, by keeping some cooked grain handy in the refrigerator.

Left over grain can be made into creamy cereals, into breads (such as the 2--slice bread - see "Breads"), salads, sauces, soups, or grain broths. Or, lightly sautée cooked grains in olive oil and garlic with freshly steamed or raw vegetables, nuts and seeds, or cooked beans or noodles. For example, see the recipe "Delicious Mixture", p.256.

Combining grains with beans and tofu, or with sauces made from beans or tofu, or with nuts and seeds increases the amino acid ratio. (See "Proteins" p.87.) For example, top your grains with a sauce made with tahini, miso or tofu (See sauce recipes.)

VARIATIONS OF INGREDIENTS IN COOKING GRAIN:

LIQUID BASES:
Cook the grain in any of the following:

    Water
    Vegetable stock
    Nut milk (See "Beverages")
    Soy milk
    Vegetable juice
    Miso stock (See "Soups")
    Herb tea (Cooking grains in teas such as
        peppermint, oatstraw or chamomile may
        aid in the digestion and assimilation
        as well as adding a different flavor.)

 MIX TOGETHER BEFORE COOKING:

    Different types of grains that have similar
        cooking time
        Good combinations are:
        rye + rice        rice + wheat
        rye + oats        rye flakes + oat flakes
        rye + barley      rice + millet
    Wheat germ
    Nuts and seeds, ground or whole
    Rehydrated (soaked) dried fruit

ADD TO COOKED GRAINS AFTER COOKING FOR TASTE
& NUTRITIONAL VARIATION:

    Steamed or raw vegetables
    sautéed onions, scallions, leeks or garlic
    soaked seaweed
    ground nuts and seeds
    cooked noodles
    cooked beans
    sprouts

## ADD TO COOKED GRAINS, CONT.:

Sauce: tofu, tahini-ginger, "super sauce",
  miso/tahini, tomato, etc. (See "Sauce"
  recipes, p.207.)
butter or butter and soy sauce
soy sauce
nutritional yeast
cayenne pepper
chopped parsley
minced ginger
spices and herbs. Whole cloves, a stick of
  cinnamon or a bay leaf can be added to
  the cooking grain to add a hint of
  flavor. Remove the herb before eating.
  Herbs and spices can be added after
  cooking, as well.
vanilla extract
honey
molasses


## GRAIN COOKING TECHNIQUES

There are several ways to cook grain,
depending on the type of grain and on the
method that is easiest for you at the time.
Whenever possible, aim for the method that
uses the lowest possible heat.

"Simmer" and "Pilaf" methods are good,
but they require the most heat.

"Soak and Simmer" or "Double boiler"
methods are better, since they use less heat.

"Soak and Steam", "Thermos" or "Quick
Steam" are best, since they require the least
amount of heat.

When you choose a method, naturally you
will need to consider what is most practical
for you as well.

PLEASE NOTE: SEE THE "GRAIN COOKING CHART" ON PAGE 251 FOR A LISTING OF GRAINS, THEIR COOKING METHODS, AMOUNTS AND COOKING TIME.

QUICK STEAM

There are two ways to quick-steam grains, depending on the type of grain.

1. For buckwheat, roasted buckwheat (kasha) and bulghur (cracked wheat):

    Put the grain in a pot.
In a separate pot, bring the liquid close to a boil, then pour it over the grain.
Stir the grain once.
Cover the pot with a tightly fitting lid.
Let stand, covered till done (about 10 to 15 minutes).

2. For rolled oats :
(Cooking buckwheat or bulghur with this method works, but the grain is a little mushy.)

    Put the grain and the liquid in a pot. Bring the liquid close to a boil. Stir the grain once. Cover the pot. Shut off the heat and let the grain cook in its own steam till done (about 10 minutes).

_____

## SOAK & STEAM

For wild rice, brown rice, barley, millet, rye, wheat, triticale:

Soak the grain in the necessary amount of liquid (see the "Chart") for 36 hours.
After soaking the grain, add more liquid, if necessary, so that you have the same amount of liquid as grain. (For example, for 1/2 c. soaked grain, you will need 1/2 c. liquid.)
Bring the soaked grain and the liquid close to a boil.
Shut off the heat.
Cover the pot and let the grain cook in its own steam for approximately 4 to 5 hours, or until done. If it is more convenient, let it steam all day, or overnight.

For example, begin to soak the grain at 8 PM Friday night. Soak time will be completed at 8 PM Sunday morning. Then let the grain sit in its own steam all day Sunday, or at least 4 to 5 hours.
Or, begin the soaking process at 8 AM Friday. Soaking will be complete 8 PM Saturday. Let the grain steam-cook overnight Saturday. It will be ready Sunday morning.

The soaked grain will keep refrigerated in its soak liquid up to one week if you do not wish to begin the steaming process right away.

## SOAK & SIMMER

For wild rice, brown rice, barley, millet, rye, wheat, triticale - whole or ground -:

12 hours before eating time, bring the grain and the liquid close to the boil, then shut the heat off, cover the pot, and let the grain cook in its own steam for 12 hours (overnight or all day).

Just before eating, bring the grain and liquid close to the boil again, turn the heat down to the lowest possible simmer, and simmer until done (about 10-15 minutes).


## THERMOS COOKED GRAIN

For wild rice, brown rice, barley, millet, whole rye, triticale. Other grains such as buckwheat, rolled oats and rye flakes can be cooked with this method but they may be too soft. Wheat cooked this way becomes rubbery. ( Note: If your thermos does not hold heat well, this technique will not work.)

Use a 1 quart wide mouthed thermos. Add the grain and any other ingredients (nuts and seeds, dried fruit, etc.), then the required amount of liquid or broth which has been heated just to the boiling point.

With the handle of a long wooden spoon, stir the grain to distribute the liquid evenly.

(Do not fill water right up to the top. Allow at least 1 inch from the top.)

Screw the lid on tightly and let stand 8 to 12 hours.

Grains can be put into the thermos whole or ground. If you want a creamy cereal, blend it after it is cooked.

## PILAF METHOD

For barley, buckwheat or kasha, bulghur, millet, oats, brown rice, wild rice, rye, triticale, wheat:

Sauté onions and/or garlic in oil in a pan that has a lid. Add the grain and, if you like, nuts and seeds. Sauté on a low heat, then add a liquid such as water, vegetable or miso stock. Cook on the lowest possible heat till nearly done, then add chopped vegetables. Cover the pan and turn the heat off so that the vegetables cook in their own steam.

## LOW SIMMER

For barley, millet, oats, brown rice, wild rice, rye, triticale, wheat:

Bring the grain and liquid close to the boil, turn the heat down to the lowest possible setting. (If possible, use a "flame tamer" between the pot and the flame.) Stir the grain once, cover the pot and let gently cook for the required amount of time. Try not to peek until the cook time is up. Otherwise, the grain tends to get mushy.

## DOUBLE BOILER

For all grains. Cornmeal, rice cream and other ground grains cook best this way.

Fill the bottom half of the double boiler about 1/3 to 1/2 full with tap water. Bring that water to a gentle simmer and leave the pot on the burner.

Meanwhile, fill the top half of the double boiler with the required amount of grain-cooking liquid and place that pot directly over another burner. Bring that liquid close to a boil, then turn it down to a gentle simmer. Slowly pour in the grain meal, stirring constantly with a wire whisk to avoid lumping. When the grain meal has absorbed the liquid, cover the pot and put it over the bottom half of the double boiler, which is still at a low simmer. Let cook till done.

If you are cooking a cereal, you can save a little time in the morning by soaking the grain overnight in the hot liquid:

Bring the ground grain (plus raisins or other dried fruit) and the liquid (water or nut milk) close to the boil, shut the heat off, cover the pot and let it sit overnight. In the morning, bring the grain and liquid close to the boil again, then put it over the double boiler and "cook" about 10 to 15 minutes.

## GRAIN COOKING CHART

| GRAIN | DRY GRAIN AMOUNT | AMOUNT OF LIQUID | QUICK STEAM | SOAK + STEAM | SOAK + SIMMER | DOUBLE BOILER | THERMOS | LOW SIMMER | PILAF | COOKED GRAIN AMOUNT |
|---|---|---|---|---|---|---|---|---|---|---|
| BARLEY | 1/2 c. | 1 1/2 c. | --- | 36+ hrs. 4 hrs. | 12+ hrs. 10 min. | 45 min. | 12 hrs. | 30 min. | 30 min. | 2 c. |
| BUCKWHEAT | 1 c. | 1 1/4 c. | 10-15 min. | --- | --- | 15 min. | 10 min. | 5 min. | 5 min. | 2 1/4 c. |
| BULGHUR | 1/2 c. | 1 c. | 10-15 min. | --- | --- | 15 min. | 10 min. | 5 min. | 5 min. | 1 1/2 c. |
| CORNMEAL* | 1/2 c. | 2 1/2 c. | --- | --- | --- | 30 min. | --- | --- | 30 min. | 3 c. |
| MILLET | 1/2 c. | 1 1/2 c. | --- | 36 hrs. 4 hrs. | 12 hrs. 10 min. | 35 min. | 12 hrs. | 20 min. | 35 min. | 2 c. |
| OATS | 1/2 c. | 2 c. | --- | 36+hrs. 5 hrs. | 12+hrs. 15 min. | 60 min. | 12 hrs. | 45 min. | 45 min. | 1 1/2 c. |
| ROLLED OATS** | 1 c. | 2 1/2 c. | 10 min. | --- | --- | 15 min. | 10 min. | --- | --- | 2 c. |
| BROWN RICE | 3/4 c. | 1 1/2 c. | --- | 36+hrs. 5 hrs. | 12+hrs. 15 min. | 45 min. | 8 hrs. | 30 min. | 30 min. | 2 c. |
| WILD RICE | 1/2 c. | 1 3/4 c. | --- | 36+hrs. 5 hrs. | 12+hrs. 15 min. | 90 min. | 12 hrs. | 60 min. | 60 min. | 2 c. |
| RICE FLOUR** | 1/4 c. | 1 c. | --- | --- | --- | 30 min. | --- | --- | --- | 2 c. |
| RYE | 1/2 c. | 2 c. | --- | 36+hrs. 5 hrs. | 12+hrs. 15 min. | 90 min. | 12 hrs. | 60 min. | 60 min. | 1 1/2 c. |
| RYE FLAKES | 1 c. | 2 1/2 c. | 10 min. | --- | --- | 15 min. | 10 min. | --- | --- | 2 c. |
| TRITICALE | 1/2 c. | 2 c. | --- | 36+hrs. 5 hrs. | 12+hrs. 10 min. | 60 min. | 12 hrs. | 45 min. | 50 min. | 1 1/3 c. |
| WHEAT | 1/2 c. | 2 c. | --- | 36+hrs. 5 hrs. | 12+hrs. 10 min. | 60 min. | --- | 45 min. | 50 min. | 1 1/3 c. |

* See "Cereals"
** Any grain can be ground to a flour and prepared as a Cream Cereal. See "Cereals".

READING THIS CHART:
This chart shows the cook time for 7 different methods of cooking grains, along with the dry grain amount, required liquid amount, and the amount of cooked grain.

******** GRAIN RECIPES ********

Note: Refer to the Index, "Grains", for other grain recipes.
   For variations in ingredients which you may add to cooked grains, and for other cooking techniques, see the introduction to this section.

## BROWN RICE (Makes 2 c. grain)

1/2 c. raw brown rice          1 c. water

Rinse the rice until the rinse water is clear. Drain. Bring the rice and water close to a boil. Turn the heat to the lowest possible setting. Stir once. Tightly cover the pot. Cook gently 1/2 hour. Try not to peek. If after the 1/2 hour, the rice is just the tiniest bit soggy, cover the pot, turn off the heat, and let sit 10 minutes. Don't stir it. It will continue to cook in its own heat.

## MILLET (Makes 2 c. cooked grain)

1/2 c. millet                  2 c. water

Rinse the millet till the rinse water is clear. Drain. Bring the millet and water close to the boil. Turn the heat to the lowest possible setting. Tightly cover the pot and cook 20 minutes.

## RICE-NUT-CHEESE LOAF (Serves 4)

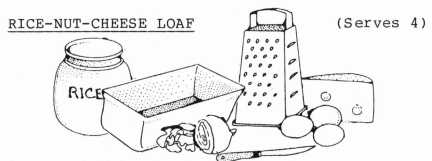

2 c. cooked brown rice
1 clove garlic, minced
1/2 c. chopped onion (1 medium sized onion)
1 c. chopped walnuts
1/4 tsp. soy sauce
2 eggs, beaten
3/4 lb. sharp cheddar cheese, grated
1/2 c. water or soy milk

Mix all ingredients. Put them into a lightly greased 9" x 5" or 10" x 6" casserole. Bake for 50 to 60 minutes at 350°. Let sit 10 minutes before cutting.
This makes a great left over - not as rich as it is when just cooked and hot.

ALTERNATE: Add 3/4 c. cooked vegetables to the other ingredients before baking. Bake as recipe is written.

## SESAME RICE (Serves 2)

2 tsp. butter          1 1/2 Tbl. sesame seeds
1/3 c. sliced leeks or scallions
2 c. cooked brown rice
Optional: 1/4 tsp. soy sauce, or to taste

Lightly sauté on a low heat the leeks or scallions, and sesame seeds in the butter. Add the rice, and stir till warm and mixed with the other ingredients. Add soy sauce to taste, if you like. This is also great with tahini gravy or "super sauce".

## PILAF CASSEROLE (Serves 3-4)

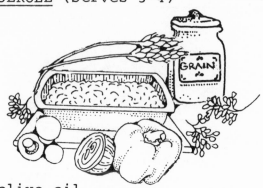

1 Tbl. olive oil
3 Tbl. chopped onion (about 1 small onion)
1/2 c. chopped mushrooms (2-3 large mush-
    rooms)
1 c. uncooked grain - bulghur, buckwheat,
    rice or millet, or a mixture of them
2 Tbl. chopped green pepper
1 Tbl. chopped parsley
1/2 c. chopped celery
1 small carrot, chopped
2 to 4 c. vegetable stock and 1 Tbl. soy
    sauce, or use miso broth (see "Soups").

Optional: add 1/2 tsp. sage or cumin

Preheat the oven to 350°.

Heat the oil in a 1 quart casserole. Lightly
sauté the onion, mushrooms, and grain, then
add the stock and any spices. The amount of
broth depends on the type of grain used in
the recipe. Refer to the suggestions on the
following page, and to the Grain Cooking
Chart to determine how much liquid to add for
the grain you choose.
Bring the liquid just to the boil, stir,
cover and reduce the heat to the lowest
possible temperature. Gently simmer 15
minutes.

Add the vegetables. Put the casserole in the oven and bake, covered, at 350° for 30-40 minutes, or until all the liquid is absorbed and the grain is dry, yet tender.

Note that this "casserole" is not meant to hold together particularly well. Rather, it is a light and fluffy mixture of grain and vegetables.

SUGGESTED COMBINATIONS FOR THE PILAF METHOD:

Following the instructions on the previous page, sauté the onion in olive oil, then add any of the following combinations and bake as indicated.:

1 c. bulghur plus sesame seeds, cumin and raisins in 2 c. vegetable stock.
(or)
1/3 c. each millet and lentils with bay leaf, sage, lovage in 4 c. vegetable broth.
(or)
1 c. brown rice plus curry powder, cumin, walnuts, bay leaf, in 2 1/2 c. water.
(or)
1 c. bulghur plus garlic and dill in 2 c. tomato juice.
(or)
1 c. brown rice plus walnuts in 2 c. miso broth.
(or)
3/4 c. millet plus 1/2 tsp. sage in 3 c. vegetable broth.

## DELICIOUS MIXTURE

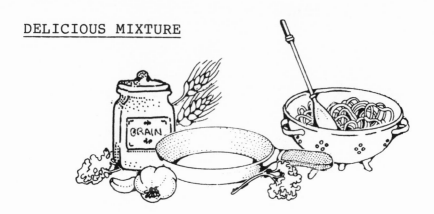

1/4 c. cooked wild rice
1/4 c. cooked Jerusalem artichoke spaghetti
   noodles
6 almonds, chopped
1/4 c. soft tofu
1 - 2 Tbl. sliced celery
2 Tbl. chopped parsley
2 Tbl. sliced green leek
1 Tbl. butter
2 tsp. soy sauce

Lightly sauté the almonds and leeks in the butter in a fry pan. Add all other ingredients and stir till warm. Add the soy sauce last, to taste.

This serves one person with a good appetite. Increase the amounts for serving more than one.

GRAIN SALADS

QUICK GRAIN SALAD (Serves 1)

Prepare 1/2 c. strong peppermint tea. While it is steeping, mix the following:

    1/2 c. bulghur (cracked wheat)
    2 Tbl. sunflower seeds
    1 Tbl. currants

Pour the tea over the above mixture and let it sit till the grain is soft (about 10 minutes). When the grain has absorbed the tea, add chopped parsley.

Note: Bulghur is wheat. If you are allergic to wheat, use unroasted buckwheat or roasted buckwheat (kasha).

Optional additions:
    These additions make the salad slightly more elaborate, but don't add that much time to the preparation.
    To the steeped peppermint tea, add:
        2 tsp. lemon juice
        1/4 tsp. cinnamon
        1/2 tsp. soy sauce

    To the salad, after soaking, add:
        1 Tbl. chopped scallions
        1/2 ripe tomato, diced

## MOCK TABOULI (BULGHUR SALAD)
(Serves between 6 and 50 people)

This is a recipe that is easy to prepare ahead for a large party. It keeps very well, up to one week refrigerated.
Also note that this recipe requires no cooking, other than boiling water!

## INGREDIENTS FOR 8 CUPS:

Combine:
    2 c. bulghur wheat
    water to cover grain (about 1 1/2 to 2 c.)
    2 peppermint tea bags
    3/4 c. sunflower seeds
    3/4 c. currants
    1/2 c. chopped parsley
    1/3 c. chopped scallions

    Optional: 1/2 c. chopped fresh mint;
        sliced tomatoes; chopped cucumber

Sauce to mix:
    1/3 c. + 1 Tbl. olive oil
    1/4 c. soy sauce     2 1/2 Tbl. lemon juice
    1/4 tsp. cinnamon    1/2 tsp.minced garlic

## INGREDIENTS FOR 50 PORTIONS:

    10 c. bulghur           3 qts. water
    6 peppermint tea bags   3 c.currants
    2 1/2 c. sunflower seeds 3 c.chop parsley
    3 c. chopped scallions  2 c.chopped mint

Sauce to mix (Make more if you prefer a more moist grain salad):
    2/3 c. lemon juice      2/3 c. soy sauce
    1 1/2 c.olive oil       1/2 Tbl.cinnamon
    3/4 Tbl. powdered garlic

MOCK-TABOULI PREPARATION:

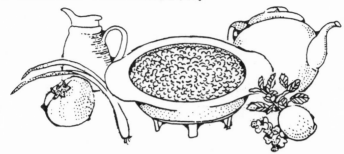

Steep the tea bags in the water until you have a strong peppermint tea.

Put the bulghur in a bowl, allowing about 3" from the top of the bowl so that the bulghur can rise as it soaks up the tea. Pour enough tea over the bulghur so that the grain is wet, but there is no tea above the level of the grain. Put a plate on top of the bulghur so that the top will not dry out. Soak for one hour, or until the grain has absorbed all the tea.

While the bulghur is soaking, put the sunflower seeds and currants in one bowl, the vegetables in another bowl, and the sauce in another bowl.

When the bulghur is soft, mix a small amount of bulghur together with small amounts of seed-currant mixture, vegetables and sauce, transferring the mixed tabouli to a separate bowl. This helps keep the tabouli light and fluffy. (This is especially necessary when making larger amounts.)
If the tabouli is drier than you prefer, add more sauce.

Decorate with cherry tomatoes, sprigs of parsley, and lettuce leaves around the edges.

## WILD RICE SALAD WITH CURRIED TOFU MAYONNAISE

(Makes 4 1/2 cups of salad)

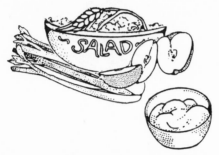

Combine:
    1 c. cooked brown rice
    1 3/4 c. cooked wild rice
    3 Tbl. slivered almonds
    3/4 c. chopped celery
    2 Tbl. chopped celery leaves
    1 Tbl. chopped parsley
    1/2 c. chopped apples

    Optional: Add 1/4 c. raisins


Curried Tofu Mayonnaise (Makes 1 1/3 c.)

Blend well in a blender till smooth:
    8 oz. firm tofu
    2 Tbl. cider vinegar
    2 Tbl. olive oil
    1/2 tsp. mustard
    1/4 tsp. soy sauce
    1 tsp. curry powder
    4 to 5 Tbl. water

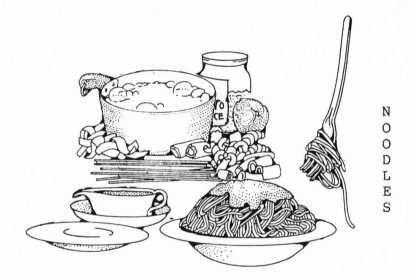

N
O
O
D
L
E
S

******** N O O D L E S ********

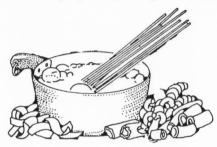

Use whole grain, unrefined, unprocessed noodles. Especially tasty are whole wheat, 100% buckwheat (which is not wheat), and those made with a combination of Jerusalem artichoke flour and whole wheat.

In general follow the cooking instructions on the package. Cook the noodles in three times the amount of liquid as the volume of noodles. Use a pot large enough to hold that amount of water without boiling over. Bring the water to a gently rolling boil, and add the noodles gradually so that the boil is not disturbed. You can hold the noodles on one end, and, while they soften, slowly push them down into the hot water.

To help keep the noodles from clumping, add a little olive oil to the cooking water. Also, to help cut the starchy covering of noodles, put the cooking water aside after you drain the noodles, rinse the drained noodles in cold water, then put them back in the cooking water for a second to re-warm them.

Noodles are a perfect food with which to experiment and create spontaneous recipes.

Noodles are delicious as a side dish with a sauce, such as the Super Sauce, p.209. Noodles are also delicious in cold salads, or added to soups, lightly sautéed vegetables, or grains.

Having noodles at the same meal with legumes (beans), or a bean by-product, such as miso or tofu, makes the usable protein more complete (See "Combining Proteins", pp.86-88.).

For other recipes that include noodles, refer to the Index, under Noodle recipes.

******** NOODLE RECIPES ********

NOODLES & SAUCE

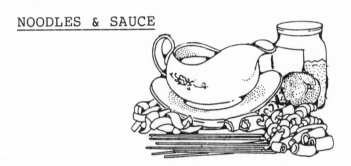

Cooked noodles are delicious with any of the following sauces or dressings:

Butter
Olive oil, minced garlic and parsley
Butter and soy sauce
Butter or olive or sesame oil and chopp-
     ed parsley
Tomato sauce (p.210)
Super Sauce (p.209)
Miso-Tahini Sauce (p.208 or 209)
Sesame Tahini Sauce (p.206)
Tahini-Ginger Dressing (p.203)
Quick Lentil Sauce (p.208)
Oil and Vinegar Dressing (p.202)
Ruth Duffy's Dressing (p.202)
Mustard Dressing (p.275)
Tofu Dressing (p.205)
Curried Tofu Mayonnaise (p.260)

## NOODLES PLUS

For an added treat, use a variety of noodles in the same dish - green or white, fettucini or shell, etc.

While the noodles are cooking, sauté on a low heat in olive oil or butter any of the following:

| | |
|---|---|
| onions | mushrooms |
| garlic | chopped leeks |
| chopped scallions | chopped peppers |
| chopped pecans, walnuts or almonds | |

Then add the noodles and any of the following:

| | |
|---|---|
| cooked grain | cooked beans |
| steamed vegetables | raw vegetables |
| chopped parsley | sprouts |
| ground or chopped nuts and seeds | |
| herbs and spices | |
| cooked chicken or fish | |

Then, if you like, top that mixture with soy sauce or any of the sauces listed above. (For example, see "Delicious Mixture" , p. 256.)

## ITALIAN TOFU AND NOODLES
(Serves 2)

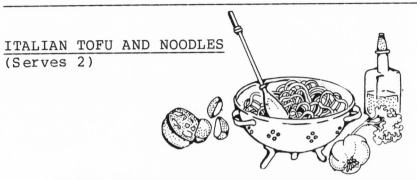

     2 oz. whole wheat/Jerusalem artichoke
       flat fettucini noodles
     1 c. tofu pieces (hard tofu, cut into
       1/2" squares)
     1 Tbl. thyme
     2 Tbl. finely chopped fresh parsley
     1 large clove garlic, minced (1 tsp.)
     1/4 c. olive oil
     1 c. chopped tomatoes

Put the noodle water on to boil.

Meanwhile, mix the thyme, parsley, garlic and olive oil in a pan that will fit under the broiler. Add the tofu pieces and stir thoroughly until the tofu is well covered with the mixture. Put the pan under the broiler to broil for 15 minutes. Stir the tofu occasionally.

By now the noodle water should be at a gently rolling boil. Put the noodles into the water and set the timer for the cook time indicated on the noodle package (usually 8 minutes). Add 1 tsp. olive oil to the water to help keep the noodles from clumping.

When the noodles and tofu are done, add the drained noodles to the pan with the cooked tofu, stirring to cover the noodles with the oil and herb mixture.

Add the chopped tomatoes and stir again. Then, if necessary, transfer the "salad" to a serving bowl.

This is delicious with a green salad, such as "Super Avocado Watercress" or "Endive Watercress". (See pp.192 and 193.)

PECAN-NOODLE SALAD (Serves 2)

    1 c. medium shell whole wheat/Jerusalem
       artichoke noodles, cooked
    1 1/4 c. sliced endive
    1 1/4 c. watercress sprigs
    14 pecans, chopped

    Blend:
    1/3 c. sesame oil
    2 Tbl. cider vinegar
    1 tsp. tarragon
    1/4 tsp. ground celery seed
    1 clove garlic, minced (1 tsp.)
    1/2 tsp. mustard

    Combine the noodles, endive, watercress
and pecans. Add about 2 Tbl. of the dressing
to the mixture, and stir thoroughly. Add more
dressing, if needed.


SUNCHOKE-NOODLES (Serves 2)

    2 oz. buckwheat noodles
    1 Tbl. sesame oil
    3 Tbl. sliced leeks
    1/4 c. slices of Jerusalem artichoke
    1/2 c. hard tofu chunks
    1/4 c. chopped parsley

    Put the buckwheat noodles on to cook.
    Put the sesame oil in a fry pan. Add the
leeks. Gently sauté, then add the sunchokes
and tofu, and stir till warm. Add the cooked
noodles and parsley. Stir again.
    Top with a quick mixture of tahini and
soy sauce, or use "Super Sauce", p.209, or
"Tahini-Ginger Sauce", p.203.

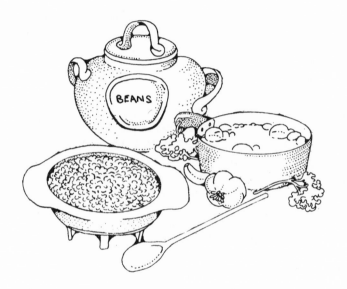

B
E
A
N
S

&

T
O
F
U

******** B E A N S  &  T O F U ********

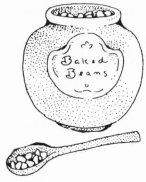

Many beans and peas can be sprouted and included in salads, or added to cooked dishes. See "Sprouts".
All beans should be rinsed in cold water until the rinse water runs clear. Remove any stones or foreign particles.

All beans, except lentils, small limas, aduki beans and split peas should be soaked for at least 3 hours before cooking.

To reduce cooking time by about 1 hour, freeze the beans overnight in fresh soak water after you have completed the 3 hour soak time. This is optional. If you do not freeze them overnight in soak water, soak and cook them for the amount of time suggested on the "Legume Cooking Chart".

Remember that beans and peas expand greatly when soaking or cooking (2 1/2 to 3 times), so use a pot, with a tight fitting lid, large enough to accomodate the increase.

For smaller beans, such as lentils, split peas and limas, use about 1/4 cup of dry beans per person for a serving. For other beans, use 1/2 c. dry beans per person.

As with grains, there are many variations in cooking liquids and in toppings for beans and peas. See next page.

For all legumes add 2-4 times more liquid than the volume of the legumes. Bring the liquid and the beans or peas just to the boil, cover the pot and turn the heat down to the lowest possible setting. Refer to the bean cooking chart, p.271, for the required amount of liquid and cooking time for each type of bean.

Beans and peas must be cooked to prevent any toxic reaction that can occur from consuming raw beans (especially raw soy beans.) However, low heat cooking is still preferable to a pressure cooker, since for most people beans will digest better if cooked on a low heat.

Some people find a crock pot works well for low heat cooking. Or, use your "flame tamer" to help you cook on a low heat and avoid burning.

To help get rid of the carbohydrate that causes intestinal gas, throw out the soak water, and add fresh water after each hour that the beans cook.

Adding a half of a potato or a teaspoon of apple cider vinegar to the cooking beans may also cut down on the gassy effect of the beans. The potato absorbs the gas-producing carbohydrate in the beans, and the vinegar aids the digestion.

Some people also report that they have less gas from beans if they eat them at the same meal with rice.

Legumes (Beans) can be eaten plain as a side dish, mixed with grains or vegetables, added to soups, or mashed as a spread or sauce. (See Quick Sauces, p.208.)

LIQUIDS IN WHICH TO COOK BEANS:

Miso stock (see"Soups")
Herb tea
Vegetable stock or juice
Water

ADD TO COOKED BEANS:

Nuts & Seeds                    chopped parsley
Onions or garlic                soy sauce
Cooked grain                    cooked noodles
Steamed vegetables              raw vegetables

Sauces or dressings, such as Tofu Sauce, Tahini Sauce, Miso/Tahini Sauce, Tomato Sauce, Curried Tofu Mayonnaise, Ruth Duffy's Tarragon Dressing. (Refer to the Index under "Dressings" for page numbers.)


SUGGESTED LEGUME (BEAN) COMBINATIONS:

(See "Legume Chart" for amounts of beans, liquid and cook time.)

* Sauté onions and garlic in olive oil, add thyme and marjoram, then lentils, tomatoes and stock. Cook on a low simmer till nearly done (about 1/2 hour) then add chopped carrots and parsley.

* Cook aduki beans and butternut squash in water. Add miso stock or soy sauce.

* Bring split peas close to a boil. Reduce heat to the lowest possible simmer, add chopped onions. Cook till nearly soft (about 25 minutes), then add chopped carrots and cook 5 more minutes.

******** LEGUME (BEAN) COOKING CHART ********

UNSOAKED BEANS (These do not need to be soaked)

| BEAN | DRY BEANS | LIQUID AMOUNT | COOK TIME | COOKED BEANS |
|---|---|---|---|---|
| Aduki Beans | 1 c. | 4 c. | 1½-2 hrs. | 2½ c. |
| Black Eyed Peas | 1 c. | 3 c. | 1 hr. | 2½ c. |
| Lentils | 1 c. | 2½ c. | 1 hr. | 3 c. |
| Split Peas | 1 c. | 2 c. | 45 min. | 2¼ c. |
| Small Limas | 1 c. | 2½ c. | 1½ hr. | 2¼ c. |

SOAKED BEANS

| BEAN | DRY BEANS | LIQUID AMOUNT | SOAK TIME | COOK TIME | COOKED BEANS |
|---|---|---|---|---|---|
| Black Beans | 1 c. | 3½ c. | 3 hrs. | 1½ hrs. | 2¾ c. |
| Chick Peas | 1 c. | 4 c. | overnight | 3 hrs. | 2½ c. |
| Great Northern | 1 c. | 2 c. | 3 hrs. | 1 hr.15 min. | 2 c. |
| Kidney Beans | 1 c. | 2 c. | 3 hrs. | 1½ hrs. | 2 c. |
| Large Limas | 1 c. | 2½ c. | 3 hrs. | 1 hr.15 min. | 2¼ c. |
| Marrow Beans | 1 c. | 2 c. | 3 hrs. | 2½ hrs. | 2 c. |
| Navy Beans | 1 c. | 3¼ c. | 3 hrs. | 1 hr.15 min. | 2½ c. |
| Pea Beans | 1 c. | 3¼ c. | 3 hrs. | 1 hr.15 min. | 2½ c. |
| Pinto Beans | 1 c. | 3½ c. | 3 hrs. | 2½ hrs. | 2 c. |
| Red Beans | 1 c. | 3 c. | 3 hrs. | 3 hrs. | 2 c. |
| Soy Beans | 1 c. | 4 c. | overnight | 3 hrs. | 3 c. |

**********

READING THIS CHART

The list of beans is divided into those that need to be soaked, and those that do not need to be soaked.

For the unsoaked beans: Bring the required amount of water and beans close to the boil. Turn the heat down to the lowest possible setting, and cook for the time indicated.

For the soaked beans: Soak them for the time indicated. Then bring the soaked beans and liquid close to a boil, turn the heat down to the lowest possible setting and cook for the time indicated.

The liquid amount indicated on this chart is based on the amount of liquid required if you cook the beans in the soak water. If, on the other hand, you throw away the soak water (to cut down on the gassy effect of the beans), measure the soak water before you throw it away, then replace with that amount of water for cooking.

For other hints on how to cut down on the gassy effect of beans, refer to the bean section.

******** LEGUME (BEAN) RECIPES ********

HUMUS (GARBANZO, OR CHICK PEA, DIP)

   2 c. cooked chick peas
   5 Tbl. Tahini (1/4 c. + 1 Tbl.)
   1/4 c. lemon juice
   2 tsp. soy sauce
   1 1/2 tsp. olive oil
   1/2 tsp. cumin (optional)
   1 Tbl. minced parsley
   2 cloves garlic, minced (about 1 tsp.)
   About 2 Tbl. chick pea cook water, or
enough so that the dip is not too thick.

Method for Cooking Chick Peas:
   1 c. dry beans = 2 to 2 3/4 c. cooked

   Soak 1 c. dry beans in 4 c. water for
2-3 hours. To help get rid of the carbohydrate in the bean that causes gas, replace
the soak water with fresh water after each
hour.
Freeze the beans in fresh soak water over
night. This will reduce cooking time. If you
do not freeze them overnight, increase
cooking time by about 1 hour.
   Bring the beans to a boil in fresh water
twice the volume of the beans. Cook on the
lowest possible simmer for 2 hours, or until
the beans are tender. You may need to add
more water after 1 hour of simmering. Be sure
that you always have enough water so that the
beans do not burn.

To make the dip:
   Put 2 cups of the cooked beans, plus all
other ingredients listed above (tahini, lemon
juice, soy sauce, olive oil, etc.) in a
blender. Blend completely. Add more chick pea
cooking water, if the dip is too thick.
   Serve with whole grain pita bread or
crackers, as a dip for raw vegetables, or as
a sandwich spread.

-272-

## LENTIL WALNUT BURGERS (Makes 4 patties)

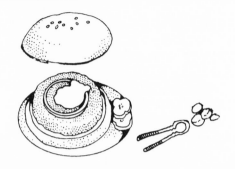

1/3 c. dry lentils
1/4 c. chopped onion
3 Tbl. chopped parsley
1/3 c. rye bread crumbs
1/3 c. chopped walnuts
1/2 to 1 tsp. thyme (1 tsp. is tasty if you like thyme.)

1 egg
1 Tbl. butter
1/2 tsp. soy sauce

Put the dry lentils in a pot with one cup of water. Bring the water close to the boil, then turn it down to the lowest possible simmer. Let cook till soft -- about 1/2 hour.

Meanwhile, chop the onion, parsley, and walnuts, and prepare the bread crumbs.

Sauté the onion in the Tbl. butter, on a low heat.

In a large bowl, mix together the walnut pieces, bread crumbs and thyme.

When the lentils are done, drain them, then put them in a blender with the sautéed onion, the soy sauce, egg and parsley. Blend till broken down, but not a liquid.

Pour the lentil mixture into the bowl of the dry mixture. Mix them together.

Form about 4 patties and put them on a lightly greased baking sheet.

Bake at 350° for 20 minutes.

Delicious hot or cold as is, or with tomato sauce, or with whole grain english muffins and sugar-free ketchup.

## WILD RICE & BEAN LOAF WITH MUSHROOM GRAVY

Loaf:
  3 eggs
  3 c. cooked navy beans
  2 c. cooked wild rice
  1 Tbl. butter
  1 medium sized onion, chopped
  1 clove garlic, minced
  1 1/4 c. chopped mushrooms
  2/3 c. chopped celery
  optional: 1 tsp. vegetable salt

Beat the eggs in a large bowl.
Add the beans and rice. Stir, then transfer
to a blender. Blend briefly so that you have
mostly "mush", with some beans and rice left
unmashed. Put the mixture back in the bowl.
Sauté the onion, garlic, mushrooms and celery
in butter. Add it to the bean/rice mixture.
(Also add the vegetable salt, if you like.)
Mix well.
Pour into a lightly greased baking pan. Bake
at 350° 30 to 40 minutes.
Top with gravy. You can use the "Super Sauce"
gravy with ginger (p.209), or the "Super
Sauce" with garlic and cumin. Or, use the
following mushroom gravy.


Mushroom Gravy (Makes 1 1/3 c.)
  1 Tbl. butter
  1/3 c. chopped onion
  1 c. chopped mushrooms
  1 c. water
  1 Tbl. kuzu
  1/4 tsp. soy sauce

Sauté the onion and mushroom in the butter.
In the blender, blend the water, kuzu and soy
sauce. Add the sautéed onion and mushroom.
Blend briefly again, then transfer back to
the sautée pan and simmer on a low heat,
stirring constantly till thick.

## BEAN SALAD WITH MUSTARD DRESSING

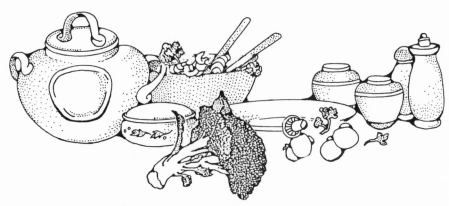

2 c. cooked Great Northern Beans
1 c. cooked green spinach macaroni (approx-
    imately 1 c. uncooked
2/3 c. sliced carrot (approximately 1 large
    carrot), raw or lightly steamed
2 stalk celery, chopped in small pieces
1 1/2 c. broccoli flowerettes, raw or
    lightly steamed
1/4 c. chopped parsley
3/4 c. sliced mushrooms

Combine the above ingredients.
Mix with the following dressing:

Mustard Dressing Makes 1/2 c.

Mix or blend well:
  2 Tbl. apple cider vinegar
  2 Tbl. mustard
  2 Tbl. tahini
  2 to 3 Tbl. water
  1/2 tsp. tarragon

ALTERNATE:
This format also makes a great chicken salad.
Use cooked diced chicken in place of cooked
beans.

## TOFU

For some people, tofu, or "soy bean curd", is a new and strange food. However, because of its bland taste, it is extremely versatile. Try incorporating it into your diet gradually, adding it to sauces (see "Tofu Dip"), soups (see "Miso Soup"), noodle dishes (see "Italian Tofu Noodle"), or grain dishes (see "Delicious Mixture"), or a dessert such as "Pineapple Tofu Custard". Or, try the following simple recipes.

For a more complete definition of tofu, see "Glossary".

SCRAMBLED TOFU
    16 oz. firm tofu, cut in small cubes
    1/4 c. chopped fresh parsley
    1 1/3 c. sliced mushrooms (about 8 large
        mushrooms)
    1/3 c. chopped red pepper
    1/3 c. chopped scallions (2 medium sized)
    1 1/2 Tbl. olive oil
    1 tsp. soy sauce
    1/4 tsp. ground marjoram
    1/4 tsp. turmeric

Sauté the scallions and mushrooms on a low heat in a large skillet. Add the remaining ingredients. Scramble gently till warm and well mixed. (3 to 4 minutes).
Add a pinch of cayenne pepper.

BROILED TOFU

Mix your favorite vegetable broth pow-der, soy sauce, water, minced garlic and ground ginger. Slice the tofu thin and dip it in the broth mixture. Marinate 1 hour or more. Place the tofu on a flat pan and put the pan under the broiler. Broil till fairly dry (about 10 minutes on a side).

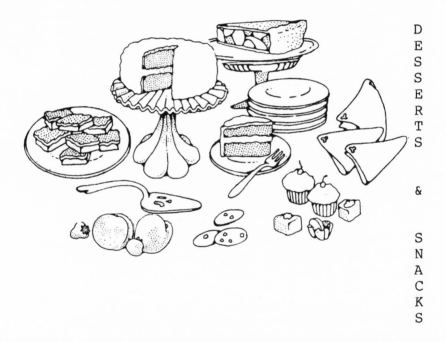

D
E
S
S
E
R
T
S

&

S
N
A
C
K
S

******** SNACKS & DESSERTS ********
RECIPES

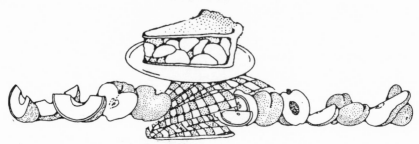

FOR MUFFINS AND DESSERT BREADS, SUCH AS
MILLET BANANA BREAD, ZUCCHINI BREAD AND
GINGERBREAD, SEE "BREADS AND MUFFINS".


## SUNNY SALTY SNACK (Makes 2 1/2 c.)

Nuts and seeds are more nutritious raw,
but this is a delicious "transition" snack.
It is a perfect holiday or "house warming"
gift, packaged in an attractive jar.

```
1 c. walnuts            1/4 c. soy sauce
1 1/2 Tbl. oil          1/8 tsp. paprika
1/4 tsp. cayenne pepper
1/4 tsp. ground celery seeds
1 c. sunflower seeds
1/2 c. pumpkin seeds
```

Put the walnuts in a shallow pan. Cover
with the soy sauce. Soak overnight.
The next day, drain the soy sauce into a
small bowl, leaving the walnuts in the pan.
Mix into the soy sauce the oil, cayenne,
paprika and ground celery seeds. Add the
sunflower seeds and mix until they are
thoroughly coated with the mixture.
Add the coated sunflower seeds to the
soaked walnuts in the shallow pan. Bake in a
preheated oven at 350° for 10 minutes.
Let cool, then mix the baked walnuts and
sunflower seeds with the pumpkin seeds.

## SNACKS TO GO

Mix any of the following to munch any time:
(Note that nuts and seeds are high in calories, and can contribute to weight gain.)

| | |
|---|---|
| almonds | sunflower seeds |
| shredded coconut | pumpkin seeds |
| soaked dried fruit | dulse |

## QUICK CANDIES (Makes 15 quarter sized, rich tasting candies)

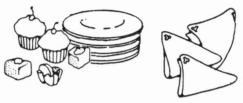

3 Tbl. ground almonds (or more, if you
plan to roll the candies in almond meal)
2 Tbl. pure carob powder
2 Tbl. tahini
4 tsp. honey, barley malt or rice bran
syrup
1 tsp. vanilla extract

Mix the ground almonds and carob powder. Add
the tahini, honey, vanilla and any flavoring
variations listed below, depending on which
taste you prefer. Mix well. Form into small
candies. Pat with ground almonds or sesame
seeds.
Note: Any time you have left over almond
meal, prepare a glass of almond milk (p.156)
to enjoy with your candies.

VARIATIONS:
For Carob Mint Kisses, add 2 drops peppermint
oil.
For carob orange candies, add 1/2 tsp. orange
extract.
For Sesame Marzipan, add 2 Tbl. shredded
coconut and 1/2 tsp. almond extract.

## SWEET TREATS

Delicious candies can be made by mixing any of the following ingredients:

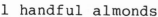

    ground or whole nuts and seeds
    rehydrated dried fruit
    sprouts
    butter
    shredded coconut
    nut butter such as almond or tahini
    unsweetened carob powder
    powdered coffee substitute
    vanilla, orange or almond extract
    peppermint, spearmint or wintergreen oil
    pure fruit juice or apple cider
    honey, maple syrup, molasses, barley malt
        or rice bran syrup


## CAROB GRAHAM CRACKERS

Put either of the following combinations of ingredients in a cuisinart or strong blender and blend to a thick paste. Add spring water if necessary:

    1 handful almonds
    2 Tbl. unsweetened carob powder
    2 Tbl. honey
    2 Tbl. butter

                        (or)

    1 handful almonds
    1 Tbl. tahini
    3 black mission figs
    3 Tbl. unsweetened carob powder
    2 tsp. honey
    1/8 tsp. vanilla extract

Spread on, or between, honey graham crackers, or rye or wheat crackers.

## CAROB BROWNIES
(Don't expect
chocolate brownies.
Do expect Delicious
carob brownies.)

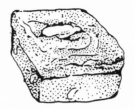

Dry Ingredients:
  1/2 c. oat flour (or) 3/4 c. rye flour
  1/2 c. carob powder
  1 tsp. baking soda
  1/2 c. filbert flour (approximately 1/3 c.
filbert nuts ground fine)
  3/4 c. chopped pecans or walnuts

  Note: If you can't find filberts, use
almonds, or an additional 1/3 c. flour. The
filberts contribute to a "chocolate" taste,
but the brownies will be good without them.
Oat flour has a more moist and chewy texture
than rye flour.

Wet Ingredients:
  3 eggs, beaten
  3/4 c. honey
  1 Tbl. molasses
  2 tsp. vanilla extract
  1/2 c. melted butter (1 stick)

Preheat the oven to 350°.
Sift together the oat or rye flour, the carob
powder and the baking soda. Stir in the
filbert flour and the chopped nuts.
In another bowl, mix the wet ingredients,
then add them to the dry. Stir till well
mixed.
Pour the batter into a lightly greased pan.
Use a 9" x 13" pan for a "chewy" texture, or
a 9" x 9" pan for a "cake" texture.
  Bake at 350° for 25 to 30 minutes.
Remove from the oven while it is still
somewhat moist in the center. It will become
more firm and dry as it cools. (It will fall
slightly.) Let cool before eating.

CAROB CHIP COOKIES
(Makes about 2 dozen cookies)

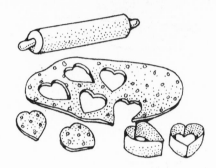

5 Tbl. butter
1 Tbl. molasses
1/2 c. honey
1/2 tsp. vanilla extract
1 c. whole wheat pastry or brown rice flour
1/2 tsp. baking soda
1 egg
1/2 c. chopped walnuts
1/2 c. unsweetened carob chips

Cream together the butter, honey and molasses.
In a separate bowl, mix the flour and baking soda.
Add the vanilla and egg to the butter mixture. Mix well, then add the flour and baking soda.
Mix well. Add the chopped walnuts and carob chips. Mix.
Refrigerate the dough 1 hour.
Lightly grease a baking sheet.
Drop the dough mixture in Tablespoon sized circles, about 1 inch apart, onto the baking sheet.
Bake in a preheated oven at 375° for 8-10 minutes.

## OATMEAL COOKIES (Makes 40 cookies)

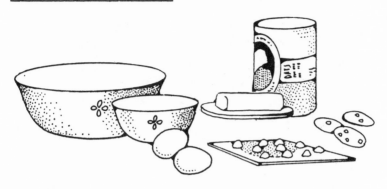

Preheat the oven to 350°.

Wet Ingredients:
  2 eggs, beaten
  1/2 c. melted butter
  1/2 c. honey or 1/3 c. barley malt
  1 tsp. blackstrap molasses
  1/2 tsp. vanilla extract

Dry Ingredients:
  2 c. rolled oats
  1/2 c. ground rolled oats
  1/4 tsp. baking soda
  1/2 tsp. cinnamon
  3/4 c. raisins
  optional: 3/4 c. chopped nuts

Beat the eggs, then add the other wet ingredients. Stir till well mixed.
In a large bowl, combine the dry ingredients.
Add the wet ingredients to the dry. Stir till well mixed.
Drop the cookie batter onto a lightly greased cookie sheet by level Tablespoons. You may need to mold them a tiny bit, if the dough doesn't hold together well.
Bake at 350° for 12-15 minutes.

## CARROT CAKE

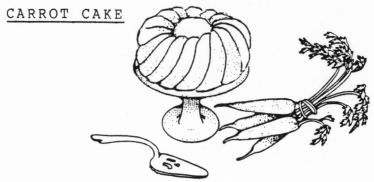

Preheat the oven to 350°.

For this recipe, use a lightly greased bundt pan, or two 9" spring form layer pans, if you wish to layer the cake. The bundt pan makes a very pretty (and delicious) cake that is great for tea time. If you use the layer pans, a lemon frosting is delicious.

Wet Ingredients:
   3 eggs
   3/4 c. honey
   1/2 c. plain yogurt
   1/2 c. melted butter
   2 c. grated carrots

Dry Ingredients:
   2 c. whole wheat pastry flour
   1 tsp. baking soda
   1 1/4 tsp. cinnamon
   (For a spicey cake, add 1/2 tsp. allspice)

In a medium sized bowl, beat the eggs, then add the other wet ingredients. Stir till well mixed.
In a large bowl, combine the dry ingredients, stirring with a wire whisk.
Add the wet ingredients to the dry, stirring till well mixed.

Pour the batter into the greased bundt pan or the layer pans.
Bake at 350° for 45 to 50 minutes.

ALMOND TORTE (Flour Free!)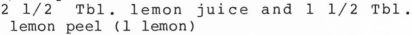

   6 egg yolks
   1/2 c. honey
   2 tsp. vanilla extract
   1/4 tsp. almond extract
   2 1/2  Tbl. lemon juice and 1 1/2 Tbl.
    lemon peel (1 lemon)
   1/4 c. cooked baking potato (about 3 oz.
    potato, skinned, diced, simmered and cool-
    ed in cold water to room temperature)
   2 c. ground unblanched almonds (1 1/2 c.
      unground. Grind 1/3 c. at a time)
   6 egg whites

Preheat the oven to 350°.
Prepare two 9" cake pans: Grease the bottoms,
but not the sides of the pans. Line the
bottoms with brown paper or parchment paper,
cut to fit. Don't grease the paper.
In a large bowl, beat the egg yolks with an
electric mixer until they are thick and lemon
colored (about 6 minutes). Add the honey, a
small amount at a time, beating another 15
minutes. Add the lemon peel, juice, and
extracts, then the 1/4 c. potato, and mix
again.
Add the ground almonds, a small amount at a
time, mixing them in very well.
In a separate large bowl, beat the egg whites
with an electric mixer until the whites form
soft peaks, but are not dry.
Gently fold the whites into the batter.
Bake 40 to 50 minutes at 350°.
Let the cake cool in the pan on a wire rack
before removing. (It will fall slightly.)
Then, carefully loosen the torte from the
sides with a knife, and remove. Let cool
before serving, or adding icing.
Serve as is, or with carob mint sauce (p.
296), kefir cheese, fresh fruit, lemon icing,
carob icing, or carob-orange icing. If you
use carob orange icing, I don't recommend
layering it, as the icing is very rich.

## BASIC VANILLA CAKE

Makes two 9" layers.

Preheat the oven to 350°.

Ingredients:
  1/2 c. honey
  6 large eggs
  1 1/4 tsp. vanilla extract
  1 1/3 c. whole wheat pastry flour
  6 Tbl. melted butter

Lightly grease two 9" layer pans, and dust them with flour.
   Melt the butter, and set it aside.
   The "secret" to this cake is mixing the eggs with an electric beater until they are high and thick. This works best if the eggs, mixing bowl and beaters are slightly warm. Simmer some water in the bottom half of a large double boiler, or any large pot. Place over the pot (but not in the water) the top of the double boiler, or any large pan or stainless steel mixing bowl.
   Pour the honey into the pot or mixing bowl, then add the eggs and vanilla. Dip the electric beaters into the simmering water to warm them.
   With the electric mixer at medium speed, beat the honey and eggs until the mixture is very thick and high, approximately 12 to 15 minutes.
   With a rubber spatula, gently fold in the flour, thoroughly mixing a small amount at a time. Then, slowly add the melted butter, thoroughly folding it in until well mixed.
   Pour the batter into the two cake pans, and bake at 350° for 30-40 minutes, or until the cake is golden brown and pulls away from the sides of the pan. Let cool on a wire rack.

Variations:
    Add the grated rind of 2 small lemons.
                    (or)
    In place of the vanilla extract, use 1
tsp. almond extract or 2 Tbl. rum.

    You could also make cupcakes out of this
batter. Fill the muffin tins 1/3 full, and
bake in a preheated oven at 375° for 20-25
minutes. Top with carob or lemon icing.


## CAKE TOPPING IDEAS

    Top each layer with carob, lemon, almond
or orange icing. (See next page.)
    Sprinkle the top with chopped or sliced
nuts; or,
    Decorate with fresh strawberries or
flowers. If you like, put a "dolop" of plain
yogurt or whipped cream or "kefir cheese"
under each strawberry.
    Cakes are also delicious with fresh fruit
in between the layers, such as mashed
rasberries.
    Or, instead of using a frosting, pour a
carob mint sauce (p.296) over a one layer
cake.

## ICINGS

    Note: "Eva's Carob Frosting" and the
"Lemon Frosting" tend to melt a bit. It
sometimes helps to put the frostings in the
refrigerator for about 45 minutes to "set"
and to put them on a cooled cake.
    It may also help to refrigerate the cake
after you have put the icing on, but before
you have smoothed the icing out on the top
and sides. (They are worth the trouble!)
    If the carob frosting is difficult to
spread, try dipping a knife in a cup of hot
water, shaking off the excess water, and
spreading the frosting with the knife.

## ICING RECIPES

### Eva's Carob Frosting:
(Makes about 1 quart, or enough for two 9"
layers.)
    1 c. honey                1 c. softened butter
    2 Tbl. vanilla extract
    1 1/2 c. unsweetened carob powder

    Stir the ingredients with a spoon till the
carob is mixed in. (Otherwise, when you turn
on the mixer, you may get a surprise
dusting.) Beat the ingredients with a mixer
until it is a frosting consistency.
    Alternate: For a delicious carob/orange
frosting, add 2 tsp. pure orange extract.

### Lemon Frosting:
    1/3 c. honey           2 Tbl. sweet butter
    Grated peel from 1 organic lemon (approx-
       imately 2 Tbl.)
    1/4 c. ground almonds

    Melt the butter on a low heat in a small
sauce pan. Meanwhile, grind the almonds in a
blender or food processor. Add the melted
butter, honey and lemon peel and blend till
well mixed.

### Almond Frosting:
    1/4 c. honey
    3 Tbl. butter, softened
    2/3 c. finely ground almonds
    1/3 c. unsweetened carob powder
    4 Tbl. cream, or 3 Tbl. kefir cheese
    1/2 tsp. almond extract

    In a medium sized mixing bowl, cream the
honey and butter. Add the ground almonds and
carob powder and mix well. Add the cream and
almond extract and beat until smooth.

## RAW FRUIT PIES

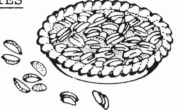

CRUST:
   3/4 lb. soft dates,
      pitted and chopped
   2 c. ground walnuts

Kneed the crust ingredients together. Press into a 10" pie plate. Refrigerate overnight to help it to harden. Fill with the "Mixed Fruit Filling".

FILLING: MIXED DRIED FRUITS:

Soak 1 cup of a mixture of dried fruit (such as apricots, prunes, pears and raisins) in the following liquid:
   1-2 c. water, or enough water so that there
      is about 1/2 inch above the fruit.
   juice of 1/2 large lemon or 1 small lemon
   1/2 tsp. cinnamon

In the morning, pour off, or strain the juice. (Save for a sauce.) Add more lemon juice and cinnamon, if you like. Put the dried fruit mixture into the pie crust. Serve as is, or chill it first.
Optional: Sprinkle with shredded coconut.

APPLE FILLING

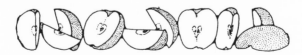

   Prepare the Raw Fruit Pie Crust, then fill with a combination of fresh apples and raisins which have been soaked overnight in lemon juice and cinnamon.

## RAW APPLESAUCE

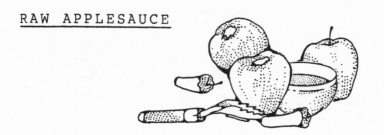

2 apples, cored and sliced in chunks
1 Tbl. raisins
1/2 tsp. cinnamon
2 Tbl. apple cider or apple juice

Optional Additions:
  1/2 banana
  dates or currants in place of raisins
  pinch of cloves

Put the apples and the juice in the blender and blend well. While blending, add the raisins and spices (and banana). Add more liquid and cinnamon, if necessary.
Serve at room temperature, or slightly warm.


## DRIED FRUIT COMPOTE

Use one or more of any of the following unsulfured dried fruit:

|          |        |         |         |
|----------|--------|---------|---------|
| apricots | pears  | prunes  | peaches |
| apples   | figs   | raisins |         |

Soak overnight in a combination of water, lemon juice and cinnamon. Use enough liquid so that there is about 1/2 inch surplus liquid over the surface of the fruit. The fruit will absorb much of the liquid and will expand. Don't cook.
Before serving, add more lemon juice and/or cinnamon to taste.

## EASY APPLE TARTS

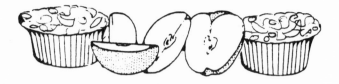

Jelled Filling (Makes 2 cups):
  1 apple, coarsely chopped
  1 1/2 c. apple juice
  2 Tbl. pure pectin
  2 1/2 Tbl. grated lemon peel
  1/2 tsp. ground cinnamon

Blend briefly in a blender so that it is
mixed, but you still have some apple chunks.
Then add and stir:
  1/3 c. raisins
Let sit in the refrigerator 2-4 hours, or
until jelled.
Note that if you just want a jello, you can
eat this as is without a crust. Put it in individual glass bowls or champagne glasses.
Sprinkle the top with grated coconut or
grated lemon peel. You can also add granola
to the jello for a crunchy texture.


Crust:
  1 c. ground granola. Grind it so that you
     still have some small chunks left.
  6 Tbl. soft butter

Preheat the oven to 350°.
Mix the ground granola and soft butter by
rubbing them in your hands. When they stick
together, line the bottom of 6 individual
baking cups with about 1/4" of the mixture.
Bake at 350° for 10 minutes. Remove the cups
from the oven and let cool at least 10
minutes.
Fill the cups with the jelled mixture.
Sprinkle with grated lemon peel.

## PINEAPPLE-TOFU CUSTARD

Blend drained tofu and drained pineapple to taste. Add honey and vanilla extract to taste.

## POPCORN, PLUS

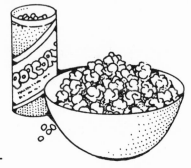

Popcorn can be a wonderful and nutritious snack. It becomes unhealthy by cooking it in oils which are too hot, which then become toxic, or by covering it with rancid oils. Popcorn is best made by using a non-aluminum screen or basket type popper, popping it dry over a hot stove or flame, or by using a non-aluminum air-type popper.

After popping, add any of the following in any combinations:

    melted butter          melted butter + oil
    soy sauce              garlic, or garlic oil
    nutritional yeast      grated parmesan cheese
    cinnamon               cayenne pepper
    vegetable salt         powdered kelp or dulse
    Dried basil + nutritional yeast, garlic
      powder and onion powder

To make garlic oil, blend, in a blender, minced garlic with a good raw olive oil.

## FROZEN FRUIT "LICK STICKS"

### FROZEN BANANAS

Peel and freeze a banana, then eat as is, or make a Carob Banana.

CAROB BANANA:
For 2-3 bananas, sliced in halves or thirds:

   1/4 c. unsweetened carob powder
   2 Tbl. water
Optional:
   vanilla or almond extract to taste

Mix the above ingredients until a thick paste. Roll the banana slices in the paste, then in the following:
   1/2 c. chopped nuts and/or shredded coconut

Put the coated banana sticks in the freezer till hard.

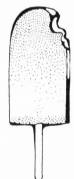

### FROZEN FRUIT STICKS

Purchase "popsicle" sticks and molds, or use small cans from frozen concentrated fruit juice. Fill the molds or cans with any of the following:

   pure juice: grape, apple, orange, pine-
     apple, papaya, mango
   peppermint tea with lemon juice and honey
   sugar-free yogurt
   layers of yogurt and fruit juice
   frozen fruit ice cream (see Recipe)
   sliced fresh fruit blended with water

Put the stick in the mold, then put the mold in the freezer till solid.

FRESH FRUIT ICE CREAM

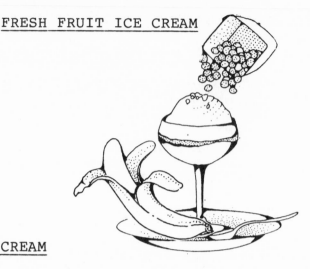

BANANA ICE CREAM

    Peel 3 ripe bananas, cut them in chunks, and put them in the freezer on a plate or wax paper. Freeze until hard, or nearly hard.
    Put the chunks, a few at a time, into a blender, food processor or champion juicer. If using a blender, you will occasionally need to stop the blender and use a rubber spatula to push the pieces down. If your blender is not too powerful, the chunks may bounce around at first. Be patient. Soon they will "catch" and become ice cream consistency. Sometimes it helps to add some unfrozen banana to the blender.

    Eat your banana ice cream plain, or with raisins, chopped nuts, carob syrup, p.296, or sliced fresh fruit.

ICE CREAM TOPPINGS

    raisins or other rehydrated dried fruit
    chopped nuts
    fresh fruit, such as peaches, blueberries,
       strawberries, rasberries
    carob sauce, p.296
    shredded coconut

## FRESH FRUIT SHERBET

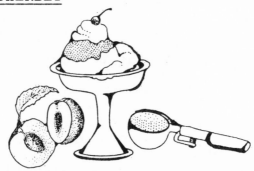

Other fruits such as peach, mango, rasberry, papaya, pineapple, blueberry, can be prepared in the same way as the banana. Peel all fruits except the berries, remove pits, and slice them in chunks. Try not to let them get too hard, as they are more difficult to blend than the banana. Their consistency will be more like a sherbet than an ice cream, unless they are combined with the frozen banana.

## FRUITY BANANA

Freeze the banana as per the Banana Ice Cream recipe. Freeze any other fruits per the Sherbet recipe, or purchase unsweetened pure frozen fruit.

Blend together an equal amount of frozen banana and any other frozen fruit. Some delicious combinations are as follows:

|                    |                       |
|--------------------|-----------------------|
| banana + peach     | banana + strawberries |
| banana + papaya    | banana + rasberries   |
| banana + mango     | banana + pineapple    |

## BANANA SPLIT

Slice unfrozen bananas and put them in a bowl. Top with fresh fruit ice cream of your choice, then with any ice cream toppings.

## QUICK DESSERT WITH CAROB MINT OR MOCHA SAUCE

Pour carob mint, mocha, orange or almond sauce over any of the following:

*   Fresh strawberries, or any other fresh fruit (kiwis, papaya, mango, peaches, pears, bananas, blueberries, apples, or any combination, such as "tropical delight", p.198).
*   Poached fruit, such as poached pear.
*   Fresh fruit ice cream or sherbet.
*   Honey Vanilla, or honey carob ice cream, or any other sugar-free, pure ice cream
*   One layer cake, such as almond torte.


### BASIC CAROB SAUCE: Makes 1 cup)

Blend in a blender:
  1/2 c. hot water
  1/2 c. honey
  1/3 c. tahini
  1 Tbl. vanilla extract
  3/4 c. unsweetened carob powder

Note that this sauce thickens in the refrigerator. You may need to add about 1/4 c. more water, in that case.

Variations:
For a carob mint sauce, add 2 drops peppermint oil. (Use a dropper.)
For a mocha sauce, add grain coffee substitute, such as pero or cafix to taste.
For a carob orange sauce, add 1 tsp. orange extract.
For an almond sauce, add 1 tsp. almond extract.
Use your own imagination, mixing the different extracts with mocha and carob, and adding the sauce to other favorite desserts.

APPENDIX

## NATURAL FOOD KITCHEN HINTS

### CLEANING VEGETABLES

Add to a sinkful of water 1 tsp. apple cider vinegar, or clorox, or wheatgrass juice. Soak fruits and vegetables (except onions) in their skins in the water for about 5 minutes. Drain and dry. This helps cut the residue of pesticides that may remain on the skin of the vegetable or fruit.

### KEEPING FOODS FRESH

GREENS:

* Keep greens refrigerated in a paper bag, rather than a cellophane one.

* Or, put any vegetables in the refrigerator vegetable bin which has been lined with paper towels or napkins. Or, put dry sponges in the vegetable bin. Any of these methods helps absorb excess moisture which rots the greens.

* To perk up wilted greens, pick off the brown edges, then sprinkle the greens with cool water. Wrap them in a paper towel and refrigerate at least one hour. Or, dip the greens in cool water to which has been added 1 tsp. lemon juice or apple cider vinegar or a few slices of raw potato. Then refrigerate.

* If you need wet greens dried quickly, put them in a pillow case and spin-dry in the washing machine.

* Keep parsley, watercress, and any fresh herbs refrigerated in a wide-mouthed glass jar with a tight lid.

* Parsley can be frozen, or can be dried by placing it on a cookie sheet in the oven with the pilot light for a few days. Store it in a glass jar after it is completely dried.

* To prevent molding of sprouts, see "Sprouts".

TOFU:
* Keep tofu refrigerated in a container of water, making sure the water covers the tofu. Change the water daily, if possible.

GRAINS, NUTS & SEEDS, FLOUR & OIL:
* Oil-base foods should be kept in the refrigerator and, whenever possible, in the freezer (particularly when there is a long storage time). This helps prevent rancidity (particularly when kept in the freezer) and bug infestation. Keeping them in glass jars is preferable since paper or cellophane bags can become soggy from melting ice.
If you buy any of these foods in bulk, keep the majority of it in the freezer, and keep smaller quantities easily available in the refrigerator.

BREADS:
* Put a stalk of celery or 1/2 apple in a bread box with the bread.
* To thaw frozen bread quickly, heat it in the oven in a brown paper bag for about 5 minutes at 325°.
* To freshen dried bread, wrap it in a damp towel, refrigerate it for 24 hours, then remove the towel and heat the bread in the oven for a few minutes.


## MISCELLANEOUS KITCHEN HINTS

TO LIQUIFY CRYSTALIZED HONEY:
* Put the honey jar in a pot of hot water and let it stand until the honey is melted.

TO HELP MEASURE HONEY:
* Lightly oil a measuring cup, or measure the oil before the honey in your recipe. The honey will easily slide out of an oiled measuring cup. Otherwise, some of it will stick to the cup and will be difficult to remove.

TO QUICKEN THE RIPENING PROCESS:
* Bury avocados in a bowl full of flour.
* Put green bananas and green tomatoes in a wet towel, then in a brown paper bag.

WHEN YOU NEED JUST A LITTLE LEMON JUICE:
* Poke a hole in the lemon, then squeeze.
* Or, slice a small piece off the end of the lemon and use that. Put the rest of the lemon in saran wrap.

STORING JARS AND LIDS
* To keep the right lid with the right jar without closing the jar (which can encourage the growth of bacteria in the jar): Hold the lid to the side of the jar with a rubber band.

## HINTS FOR EASY CLEANING OF UTENSILS

It is helpful in setting up your kitchen to keep the utensils most often used near your work space and, if possible, near the sink. For example, have a hanging rack where small utensils such as measuring spoons and cup, grater, wire whisk, etc. can drip dry.

Try to wash utensils and equipment as soon as possible after use, so that dried out food does not stick to them. If this is not convenient, put them in a sink or dish pan full of hot water until you can wash them thoroughly. Or, fill your used pots and pans and measuring cup with hot water and put the utensils in them until future washing.

Be sure to leave all blenders and juicers uncovered after washing, to air them out and help prevent the growth of bacteria.

### BLENDER:
* If it is not possible to scrub your blender right away, fill it with water and clean it later.
* Or, fill the blender half way with water and add a drop of detergent. Blend, covered, for a few seconds. Rinse and let drain dry.

### GARLIC PRESS:
* Put the garlic press in hot water right away after use, as it is difficult to remove dried pieces of garlic. If necessary, use a toothpick to remove the garlic pieces.

### GRATER:
* Use a toothbrush to remove lemon peel, onion, cheese, etc. from your grater.
* Before using the grater, rub it with olive oil to prevent food from sticking to the grater.

### CUTTING BOARD:
* To remove onion or garlic smell, cut a lemon or lime and rub the board with the cut end of the fruit.

# SECTION IV, APPENDIX - COMMON FOOD ADDITIVES

## COMMON FOOD ADDITIVES

This list, comprising the additives most commonly listed on packaged foods, is to assist you in reading labels. * Doctors recommend avoiding the additives with an asterisk.

| NAME | FUNCTION | USED IN | LEVEL OF TOXICITY |
|---|---|---|---|
| Agar (A carbohydrate extracted from seaweed) | Prevent icing from drying out. Gelling ingredient. | Cup cakes | Non-toxic |
| *Artificial Color and Artificial Flavor | Used to entice consumer to buy the product. | Commercially packaged cereals, candy, jams, ice cream, cheese, baked goods, butter, dessert powder, fruit skins (such as lemon and orange), packaged sausage. | No nutritive value. Disguises lack of nutritious ingredients, and age. Color: Coal tar dyes are suspected carcinogens (cancer causing substances). Insufficient testing has been done. However, increasing tests show high levels of toxicity in the dyes. Flavor: Little testing has been done. |
| *Benzoic Acid | Flavor preservative and anti-mold ingredient. | Jams, jellies, beverages, candies. Also used in ice for cooling fish. | Toxic. Tests on humans showed irritation to eyes, skin and mucous membranes. Tests on rats resulted in retarded growth, brain damage and possibly cancer. |
| Brominated Vegetable Oil | Used to make the oils look cloudy, which gives the appearance of thickness. | Oils | Insufficient testing. Some studies have shown harmful effects to animal's heart, kidneys, liver, thyroid and testicles. |
| *BHA (Butylated Hydroxyanisole) and BHT (Butylated Hydroxytoluene) | Anti-oxidants; that is, prevents polyunsaturated oils from oxidizing and becoming rancid. | Cake mixes, cereals, breads, crackers, dry soups, pork, instant teas, vegetable oils, steak sauces | Toxic. Tests done on rats showed that their cholesterol levels rose, hair fell out, and they were born without eyes. |
| *Calcium Disodium EDTA (Ethylenediamine tetraacetate) | Helps promote and retain color, flavor and texture. | Soft drinks, canned vegetables, sauces, spreads, dressings. | Toxic. Tests on humans resulted in kidney damage, vitamin and mineral imbalance, gastro-intestinal distress and muscle cramps. |

-302-

| | For flavor and color | | |
|---|---|---|---|
| Caramel | | instant teas, bread, soft drinks, candies | Being tested by FDA. Possibly toxic. |
| Carrageenan, or "Irish Moss" (A seaweed extract) | Suspending agent, stabilizer, thickener, emulsifier, gelling ingredient. | Chocolate drinks, soft drinks, fruit juices, milk alcohol, vinegar, products & cheese, frozen desserts, soups, sauces, dressings, canned meats, baked goods. | Non toxic, although tests with large amounts showed ulcers in animals. Low dosages have been used for medicinal purposes. |
| Citric Acid | Anti-oxidant. Prevents spoilage and discoloration of food. Adds a tart flavor. | Jellos, juices. | Safe. |
| Dextrose | Sweetener | Canned soups, dressings. | Toxic as any sugar. |
| "Enriched" | To increase the nutrient value of the product, thereby simulating a "nutritious" product to the consumer. | Breads, noodles | Non-toxic, but little nutritional value compared to the unprocessed grain. 3 or 4 synthetic vitamins and minerals, such as iron, and 3 of the B complex vitamins (thiamin, riboflavin and niacin) are added to a product which, through the refining process, has been stripped of at least 25 of its original nutrients. |
| Gums: Arabic, Ghatti, Karaya, tragacanth, xanthan | Improve texture (as in ice cream), prevent sugar from crystallizing; stabilize foam in beer; hold flavor in drink mixes, thickener | Candy, beer, ice cream, powdered drink mixes, colas. | Insufficient testing. May cause allergic reactions such as diarrhea or constipation. |
| Hydrolyzed Vegetable Protein (or protein hydrolysate) | Flavor enhancer | | Toxic. Contains MSG (See MSG). Tests showed damage to brains of infant mice. |

COMMON FOOD ADDITIVES, CONT.

| NAME | FUNCTION | USED IN | LEVEL OF TOXICITY |
|---|---|---|---|
| *Modified Food Starch | Binder, filler, stabilizer; makes the food resistant to high temperature and helps prevent doughy, rough or watery textures. | Bread, baked goods, baby food, soups, sauces, pie fillings, prepared dinner products, frozen pizza, frozen fish, canned corn, dry roasted nuts | Being tested. Nutritionally worthless, often replacing more nutritious ingredients. Tests on humans indicate that they are difficult to digest, and may raise blood cholesterol levels. |
| Mono- and Diglycerides | Prevents oil from separating; makes cakes and breads soft and keeps them from becoming stale, by preventing starch from crystalizing | peanut butter, cup cakes, bread, margarine, broths, shortenings | Being tested by FDA. May cause birth defects, genetic changes, cancer. |
| *MSG (Monosodium glutamate) | Flavor enhancer and appetite stimulator | soups, sauces, salad dressings, processed cheese, Chinese food, dry roasted nuts, canned meats, frankfurters, frozen pizza | Toxic. Can cause headaches and tightness of chest. Lab tests on mice revealed brain damage, damage to the retina of the eye, and injury to the mice fetus. |
| "Natural Sweeteners" | To sweeten a product. |  | Chemically refined cane juice. A toxic sugar. |
| Propionates - Calcium or Sodium | To prevent the growth of mold and certain bacteria. | Breads | In general, the propionates are harmless, although some studies indicate allergic reactions, with symptoms of headaches and gastro-intestinal stress similar to a gall bladder attack. |
| Propyl Gallate | Preservative | Vegetable oils and shortenings, chewing gum, pickles | Still being tested. Possibly toxic. May cause liver damage, birth defects. |
| *Propylene Glycol Alginate | Thickener, stabilizer, solvent | soft drinks, jelly, mustard, potato chips, crackers, cream cheese, yogurt, ice cream, frozen desserts | Being investigated by FDA. Glycol is used as an anti-freeze. Substances in this additive are used for anti-freeze, oils and waxes. |
| *Red Dye 40 | Food coloring to entice the consumer | red pistachio nuts, chewing gum, candies, frankfurters | Toxic. May be cancer-causing and cause birth defects. |

| Additive | Purpose | Found In | Effects |
|---|---|---|---|
| *Saccharin | To sweeten in place of sugar, since it costs the manufacturer 1/20th as much as sugar and is 300 to 500 times sweeter. | soft drinks, colas, puddings, powder mixes | Still being tested. Probably a carcinogen (cancer causing substance) |
| *Sodium Erythorbate | Preservative | Many baked goods and beverages, bacon, frankfurters | Toxic. Banned in several countries. May cause genetic defects. |
| *Sodium Nitrate and Sodium Nitrite | Prevent the growth of bacteria that causes botulism. Improves color in meat by causing the pigment to turn red. | Packaged meats (bologna, salami, ham, corned beef, pastrami, etc.), sausage, frozen pizzas. | Disguises age and poor quality of meat. Nitrites can lead to the formation of nitrosamines, proven cancer-causing substances. Under certain conditions, nitrates will become nitrites. |
| *Sulfur Dioxide | Preservative, anti-oxidant and anti-browning agent. | Wine, corn syrup, dried fruit, glaceed fruit, imitation jelly, maraschino cherries. | Toxic. Tests on humans showed symptoms of nausea, headaches, listlessness, anemia, increased uric acid, destruction of blood corpuscles. |

******** HIDDEN SUGARS ********

The following chart shows approximately how many teaspoons of sugar are added to certain food items. In addition to these, sugar is added to breakfast cereals (Some have more sugar than grain!), and many other canned and processed foods. Read labels. Keep in mind that 3 tsp. sugar = 385 calories.

| FOOD | AMT. | APPROX.# TSP.SUGAR | FOOD | AMT. | APPROX.# TSP.SUGAR |
|---|---|---|---|---|---|
| **BEVERAGES** | | | **CAKES, COOKIES & PASTRIES** | | |
| Soft Drinks | 8 oz. | 5 | Average cakes | | |
| Cordials | 3/4 oz. | 1½ | & pastry | 4 oz. | 4-6 |
| Hi-Ball | 6 oz. | 2½ | Iced chocolate cake | 4 oz. | 10 |
| Whiskey Sour | 3 oz. | 1½ | Iced cup cake | 1 | 6 |
| Sweet Cider | 1 c. | 6 | Strawberry | | |
| Sweetened Canned | | | shortcake | 1 piece | 4 |
| Fruit Juice | 1/2 c. | 2 | Plain donut | 1 | 3 |
| | | | Glazed donut | 1 | 6 |
| **DAIRY PRODUCTS** | | | Hamburger bun | 1 | 3 |
| Ice cream | 1/3 pt. | 3½ | Unfrosted brownie | 3/4 oz. | 3 |
| Ice cream bar | 1 | 1-7 | Chocolate cookie | 1 | 1½ |
| (Depending on size) | | | Fig newton | 1 | 5 |
| Ice cream cone | 1 | 3½ | Ginger snap | 1 | 3 |
| Ice cream soda | 1 | 5 | Macaroon | 1 | 6 |
| Ice cream sundae | 1 | 7 | Nut cookie | 1 | 1½ |
| Sherbet | 1/2 c. | 6 | Oatmeal cookie | 1 | 2 |
| Malted milk | | | Sugar cookie | 1 | 1½ |
| shake | 10 oz. | 5 | Chocolate eclair | 1 | 7 |
| | | | Cream puff | 1 | 2 |
| **CANDIES** | | | Brown Betty | 1/2 c. | 3 |
| Chocolate bar | 2 oz. | 8 | Pies:apple,lemon | | |
| Chocolate mint | 1 | 2 | peach,apricot: | 1 piece | 7 |
| Fudge | 1 oz. | 4½ | berry, cherry: | 1 piece | 10 |
| Gum drop | 1 | 2 | | | |
| Hard candy | 4 oz. | 20 | **CONDIMENTS** | | |
| Life savers | 1 | ½ | Ketchup | 1 Tbl. | 1 |
| Peanut brittle | 1 oz. | 3½ | Jams & Jellies | 1 Tbl. | 4-6 |
| Chewing gum | 1 stick | ½ | Apple or Peach | | |
| | | | Butter | 1 Tbl. | 1 |
| **MISC. DESSERTS** | | | | | |
| Canned apricots: | | | **SYRUP, SUGARS & ICINGS** | | |
| 4 halves & 1 Tbl.syrup | | 3½ | Chocolate or white | | |
| Canned peaches: | | | icing | 1 oz. | 3½ |
| 2 halves & 1 Tbl. syrup | | 3½ | Chocolate sauce | 1 Tbl. | 3½ |
| Canned fruit | | | Canned fruit | | |
| salad | 1/2 c. | 3½ | syrup | 2 Tbl. | 2½ |
| Canned stewed | | | | | |
| fruit | 1/2 c. | 2 | Actual sugar content of the | | |
| Jello | 1/2 c. | 4½ | following: | | |
| Chocolate pudding | 1/2 c. | 4 | Corn syrup | 1 Tbl. | 3 |
| Date or fig | | | Karo syrup | 1 Tbl. | 3 |
| pudding | 1/2 c. | 7 | Brown sugar | 1 Tbl. | 3 |
| plum pudding | 1/2 c. | 4 | Granulated sugar | 1 Tbl. | 3 |
| rice pudding | 1/2 c. | 5 | Maple syrup | 1 Tbl. | 5 |
| tapioca pudding | 1/2 c. | 3 | Molasses | 1 Tbl. | 3½ |
| banana pudding | 1/2 c. | 2 | Honey | 1 Tbl. | 3 |
| sherbet | 1/2 c. | 9 | | | |

******** HIDDEN SALT ********

The following chart shows the sodium content in common and processed foods. Note the difference between fresh and canned vegetables.

| FOOD | FOOD AMT. | APPROX.MG. OF SODIUM |
|---|---|---|
| **CAKES,COOKIES,SNACKS** | | |
| Cheese crackers | 10 | 325 |
| Ritz crackers | 9 | 288 |
| Corn chips | 1 oz. | 231 |
| Potato chips | 10 | 200 |
| Pretzels | 10 | 1,008 |
| Pillsbury sugar cookies | 3 | 210 |
| Hostess Twinkies | 1 | 240 |
| Popcorn,salted | 1 c. | 180 |
| Popcorn,unsalted | 1 c. | 1 |
| Sweet roll | 4"round | 240 |
| Doughnut | 1 | 160 |
| McDonald's apple pie | 1 | 414 |
| Peanut brittle | 1 oz. | 145 |
| Peanuts,salted | c. | 275 |
| Peanuts,unsalted | c. | 2 |
| | | |
| **BREADS & CEREALS** | | |
| Oatmeal,salted | 1 c. | 520 |
| Kellogg's All Bran | c. | 370 |
| Rice Crispies | 1 c. | 280 |
| Puffed wheat, puffed rice, | | |
| shredded wheat | 1 c. | 1 |
| Corn flakes | 1 c. | 165 |
| Bran flakes | c. | 340 |
| Bread | 1 slice | 130 |
| | | |
| **DAIRY PRODUCTS** | | |
| Butter,Margarine, | | |
| salted | 1 Tbl. | 140 |
| unsalted | 1 Tbl. | 1 |
| Low fat milk/yogurt | 1 c. | 120 |
| Buttermilk | 1 c. | 275 |
| Cottage cheese, | | |
| creamed | c. | 180 |
| unsalted | c. | 30 |
| Parmesan cheese | 1 Tbl. | 40 |
| American cheese | 1 oz. | 320 |
| Cheddar,Muenster, | | |
| Swiss cheese | 1 oz. | 220 |
| Low fat cheese | 1 oz. | 200 |
| | | |
| **PHARMACEUTICALS** | | |
| Alka Seltzer | 1 dose | 521 |
| Bromo Seltzer | " | 717 |
| Brioschi | " | 710 |
| Miles Nervine | " | 544 |
| Fleet's Enema | " | 300 |
| Metamucil Instant Mix | " | 250 |
| Rolaids | " | 53 |

| FOOD | FOOD AMT. | APPROX.MG. OF SODIUM |
|---|---|---|
| **SOUPS,BEVERAGES** | | |
| Soup,homemade,salted | 1 c. | 500 |
| commercial,canned | 1 c. | 760 |
| Instant broth mix | 1 packet | 818 |
| McDonald chocolate shake | 1 | 328 |
| | | |
| **MEATS** | | |
| Beef,Veal | 3 oz. | 75 |
| McDonald's Big Mac | 1 | 1,510 |
| Chef Boyardee Beefaroni | 7.5oz. | 1,186 |
| Ham,cured | 3 oz. | 675 |
| Ham,uncured | 3 oz. | 560 |
| Bacon | 1 slice | 75 |
| Canned Franks/Beans | 8 oz. | 958 |
| Lamb,pork,chicken | 3 oz. | 75 |
| Frozen fried chicken | 1 dinner | 1,152 |
| Frankfurter | 1 | 540 |
| Bologna | 1 slice | 390 |
| Canned tuna fish | 3 oz. | 430 |
| Fresh fish(except shell) | 3 oz. | 75 |
| | | |
| **VEGETABLES & BEANS** | | |
| Asparagus,fresh | 6 spears | 4 |
| canned | 6 spears | 410 |
| Peas,fresh | 3 oz. | 2 |
| canned | 3 oz. | 236 |
| Green Beans,fresh | 1 c. | 5 |
| canned | 1 c. | 925 |
| Corn,fresh | 1 c. | 5 |
| canned | 1 c. | 500 |
| Dry beans,unsalted | c. | 15 |
| salted | c. | 350 |
| | | |
| **MISCELLANEOUS** | | |
| Jello,instant | c. | 404 |
| Peanut butter,processed | 2 Tbl. | 172 |
| Homemade,unsalted | 2 Tbl. | 36 |
| Ice cream | c. | 42 |
| Green olive | 1 | 155 |
| Dill Pickle | 1 large | 1,400 |
| Miso | 1 Tbl. | 500 |
| Soy Sauce | 1 Tbl. | 1,300 |
| Salt | 1 tsp. | 2,300 |
| Commercial dressing | 1 Tbl. | 200-300 |
| McDonald's Egg McMuffin | 1 | 914 |
| Worcestershire sauce | 1 Tbl. | 315 |
| Frozen Pizza | 2 oz. | 328 |
| Commercial ketchup | 1 Tbl. | 200 |
| Commercial mustard | 1 Tbl. | 212 |
| Processed baby food | 3 oz. | 293-510 |

******** QUICK PLANNED MENUS ********

These menus include quick recipes, and illustrate simple preparation techniques that are suggested in this book. See "Notes for Planned Menu Chart". Wait 1 to 1½ hours before dessert to aid digestion.

| BREAKFAST | LUNCH | DINNER |
|---|---|---|
| Green drink<br>Oatmeal with nut milk<br>Special calcium tea | Raw vegetables with tofu dip<br>Quick grain salad | Quick parsnip soup<br>Sunburgers<br>Salad with quick carrot dressing<br>Dessert: Zucchini Bread |
| Green drink<br>2 poached eggs on steamed broccoli<br>Essene bread | Quick split pea soup<br>Sunburgers<br>Green salad | Quick fish<br>Sesame rice<br>Salad with mixed vegetables<br>Dessert: Carob chip cookies |
| Buckwheat cereal with nut milk<br>Millet/banana bread<br>Tea: Mint refresher | Lemon-Egg Soup with rice in it<br>Sauerkraut<br>Quick 2-Slice Buckwheat bread | Quick potato soup<br>Tomato-zucchini saute<br>Quick avocado/watercress salad with lemon/soy dressing<br>Dessert: Apple sauce |
| Green drink<br>2 soft boiled eggs<br>Essene bread with honey-carrot marmalade | Quick gaspacho soup<br>Rice cake with miso/tahini spread and sprouts | Quick miso soup<br>"Delicious mixture" (wild rice and noodle saute)<br>Salad<br>Dessert: "Sweet Treats" candies |
| Super cereal with nut milk<br>Rye/Carrot muffin<br>Herbal tonic tea | Wild rice salad<br>Raw vegetables with tofu dip | Lentil tomato soup<br>Pecan/noodle salad<br>Dessert: Banana ice cream |
| Breakfast-in-a-Glass | Pecan noodle salad<br>Rice with lentil sauce | Quick borscht<br>Lentil walnut burgers<br>Millet<br>Dessert: Fresh fruit pudding |
| Cream of millet cereal with nut milk, soaked currants and sliced banana<br>Calcium tea | Baked chicken<br>Salad | Curried chicken<br>Salad<br>Dessert: Pineapple tofu custard |

---

**** NOTES FOR PLANNED MENU CHART ****

The suggested menus on this chart are quick, delicious and nutritionally well balanced. They incorporate simple menu planning and preparation ideas, and time saving techniques that are covered in this book, such as:

1. <u>PROTEIN COMBINING</u>
Combining any of the following categories of foods makes a whole protein, when eaten within 16 hours.:
Seeds and nuts  +  Legumes, such as:
     lentil-walnut burgers
     miso-tahini spread
     sunburgers + split pea soup
     pecan noodle salad + lentil soup or lentil sauce
Legumes  +  Grains, such as:
     tofu dip + grains   (or)       miso soup + grain
     miso/tahini spread + rice cake
     lentil sauce + rice
Seeds and Nuts  +  Grains, such as:
     nut milks on cereal

2. <u>MAKING QUICK BLENDED SOUPS</u>, such as:
quick gaspacho;  quick parsnip soup;  quick potato soup

3. <u>USING LEFT-OVERS CREATIVELY</u>
Use left over grain for a creamy cereal the next day, or for a soup or salad such as:
     cream of millet cereal
     wild rice salad
     lemon-egg soup which has rice in it
Use left over beans in a soup, salad, or sauce, such as:
     lentil sauce
Make enough burgers so you have left overs for another meal, such as:  lentil-walnut burgers; sunburgers

4. <u>PRE-PREPARED DIP</u>
Make a great dip to use with vegetables, grains, beans, etc. Add water to it to make a sauce. For example:
  miso-tahini spread     tofu dip     tahini dip

5. <u>AVOIDING POOR COMBINATIONS</u>
Avoid combinations, such as protein + fruit, or protein + starch, with a few exceptions, such as fish + rice; banana + millet (or)  eggs + essene bread.

6. <u>TO HELP AVOID FRESH VEGETABLE WASTE</u>
If you have more vegetables than you need for 1 meal, plan another meal soon after which incorporates the same vegetables. For example:
  tomato zucchini sauté at one meal
  quick Gaspacho soup, using tomatoes and zucchinis

---

7. <u>MOST IMPORTANT, USE THESE TIPS TO CREATE YOUR OWN RECIPES THAT ARE QUICK, DELICIOUS AND FULL OF HEALTH.</u>

******** BREAKFAST MENU SUGGESTIONS ********

Breakfast suggestions are listed by food category, since breakfast normally consists of one main course. See "Planning Meals" for key considerations in creating a menu.

Don't limit your tastes for breakfast ideas. Try having fish, salad, - any "substantial" food you enjoy.

Having protein, a salad and fresh vegetable juice for breakfast can help sustain energy throughout the day, much better than something sweet such as pancakes or cereal with dried fruit.

## CEREALS
Top with nut milk (pp.154-156), soy milk, grain water (pp.166-167) or pure fruit juice, such as apple or pineapple.

Cream of grain, pp.134,135          Oatmeal, p.133
Super Cereal, pp.138-39             Cornmeal Cereal, p.136
Millet, p.135  Buckwheat, p.134      Granola,p.140

## FRUIT
Raw apple sauce, p.290              Raw fruit pie, p.289
Avocado and pink grapefruit, p.198
  with poppy seed dressing, p.204
Tropical delight, p.198
  with Quick Fruit Dressing, p.201

## EGGS
Poached, p.146                      Soft boiled, p.146
Fried, scrambled or omelette, p.147

## PANCAKES
Potato pancakes, p.238              Buckwheat Pancakes, p.142
Cornmeal Pancakes, p.143

## BREADS
Top whole grain toast or English muffins, or the breads or muffins listed below with strawberry jam (p.212); honey-carrot marmalade (p.212); raw honey; barley malt; unsalted dairy butter; kefir cheese, goat cheese, almond butter; tahini; miso-tahini spread (p.208 or 209); or a mixture of tahini plus honey or barley malt with cinnamon.

Essene bread, p.121                 Rye bread, p.122
Zucchini bread, p.125               Corn muffins, p.127
Millet-banana bread, p.124          2-Slice bread, p.123
Applesauce muffins, p.128           Gingerbread, p.126

BREAKFAST SUGGESTIONS, CONT.

BLENDER DRINKS
Sunflower almond milk, p.156       Almond milk, p.156
Mixed vegetable juice, p.160-161  Sesame milk, p.156
Pineapple green drink, p.162       Protein punch, p.162
Banana smoothies, p.158-159        Tofu malt, p.159
Fenugreek fluff, p.159             Brilliant Mary, p.161

BREAKFASTS IN A GLASS:
Sunflower egg, p.157  Cherry egg, p.157  Egg nog, p.157
Pineapple green drink with egg added, p.162

HERB TEAS
Mint refresher, p.169  Tummy Soother, p.169
Special calcium tea, p.169

SOUPS
Having soups for breakfast often sustains the energy throughout the day better than cereals. Have a piece of bread, toast or muffin with your soup. (See previous page for a list of breads and muffins.)
One delicious combination with vegetable or fish soup is rye toast topped with miso/tahini spread and chopped watercress leaves.
Miso Fish Soup, p.179         Miso Tofu Soup, p.179,182
Vegetable Soup, p.179,180  Pumpkin Soup, p.186
Potato Peeling Broth, p.170

SALADS
Avocado/Watercress, p.192
Raw Vegetables, p.194
    with Tofu Dip, p.205
    (or) Guacamole, p.205
    (or) Spring Green Dip, p.206.

OTHER IDEAS
Scrambled tofu, p.276
One-half small avocado, or one-quarter large avocado,
    with lemon juice and soy sauce
Sweet potato pudding, p.237

******** LUNCH OR DINNER SUGGESTIONS ********

Lunch and dinner suggestions are listed within menus
in order to give you ideas of different combinations. Experiment according to your own needs and taste preferences.

### CHICKEN

* Curried chicken, p.216
  Raw vegetables, p.194  with Spring Green Dip, p.206
  Pure mango-chutney (store bought)
  Pineapple-papaya ice cream, p.294

* Chicken Noodle Soup, p.179
  Green Salad with Watercress Dressing, p.203
  Corn Muffins, p.127

* Coq au Vin, p.215
  Steamed green peas with slivered almonds
  Salad with Mustard Dressing, p.275
  Carob Mint Kisses, p.279

* Quick Squash Soup, p.176
  Chicken & Sunchoke Noodles, p.227 (Create-A-Meal)
  Green Salad
  Applesauce, p.290

* Chicken Salad, p.191
  Spinach Salad (spinach, mushrooms and scallions)
  Quick 2-Slice Bread, p.123

### FISH

* Artichoke, p.239
  Quick fish, p.219
  Pea salad, p.194
  Fresh strawberries with carob sauce, p.296

* Fish orientale, p.220
  Sesame rice, p.260
  Salad with Oil & Vinegar Dressing, p.202
  Carrot cake, p.284

* Poached Fish, p.227 (Create-A-Meal)
  Steamed Broccoli and Leeks
  Quick 2-Slice Bread, p.123

* Quick Sweet Potato Soup, p.176 or 186
  Ginger Fish and Noodles, p.227 (Create-a-Meal)
   with Super Sauce, p.209
  Green Salad with oil and lemon juice
  Apple Tart, p.291

* Fish 'n Rice, p.227 (Create-A-Meal)
  Avocado Sunchoke Salad, p.193

* Miso Fish Soup, p.179 (Create-A-Soup)
  Baked Squash, p.236
      with Gingered Carrot Marmalade, p.212
  Spinach Salad with Mustard Dressing, p.275
  Almond Torte, p.285, with lemon frosting, p.288

* Tomato Fish Soup, p.179 (Create-A-Soup)
  Kasha, p.134 (or see Grain Cooking Chart, p.251)
  Green Salad with Carrot Ginger Dressing, p.203

* Guacamole, p.205
  Broiled fish in lemon sauce, p.220
  Brown rice, p.252, with miso-tahini sauce, p.208 or 209
  Honey carob ice cream with carob mint sauce, p.296

## VEGETARIAN

* Lentil-Tomato soup, p.177 or 183
  Raw vegetables, p.194 with Tahini dip, p.206
  Popcorn, p.292

* Raw spinach soup, p.185
  Marinated vegetables, p.195
  Salad with Sunflower-beet dressing, p.202

* Quick parsnip soup, p.176
  Sauerkraut, p.196
  Rice cakes with miso-tahini spread, p.208
      and sprouts, store bought, or see p.109

* Pumpkin Soup, p.186
  Avocado and Watercress Salad with tofu & sunchokes
      topped with lemon juice & soy sauce, p.192
  Quick 2-Slice Bread, p.123, with Miso/Tahini Spread,
      p.208 or 209

* Vegetable soup, p.179 or 180
  Herbed Potato, p.242
  Avocado/watercress salad with tamari dressing, p.192

* Raw vegetables, p.194, with Spring green dip, p.206
  Cranberry relish, p.212
  Essene bread, p.121

* Whole grain spaghetti noodles with tomato sauce, p.210
  Mixed Salad with oil and vinegar dressing, p.201 or 202
  Banana Split, p.294

* Delicious mixture  (noodles, rice and vegetables),p.256
  Alfalfa croquettes, p.195
  Sesame Marzipan, p.279

* Spicey Soba (Create-A-Meal), p.227
  Green Salad with lemon juice
  Carob Graham Crackers, p.280

* Carrot Salad, p.191
  Fermented seed loaf, p.234, in red pepper shell with
     watercress sprig on top
  Green salad with watercress dressing, p.203

* Buckwheat-sunchoke noodles, p.266
     with Super sauce, p.209
  Steamed garlic broccoli, p.239
  Salad with Quick Carrot Dressing, p.201
  Pineapple Tofu Custard, p.292

* Raw vegetables with tofu dip, p.205
  Broccoli quiche, pp.232-233
  Green salad with sunflower beet dressing, p.202
  Zucchini bread, p.125

* Rice-cheese-nut loaf, p.253
  Watercress Endive Salad, p.193,
     with Tarragon Dressing, p.202
  Mint Refresher Tea, p.169

* Miso soup, p.182
  Whole grain noodles and brown rice, p.252
     with Tahini-Ginger sauce, p.203
  Salad
  Corn muffins, p.127

* Onion soup, p.181
  Tomatoes provincale, p.237
  Mixed Green Salad with Oil & Vinegar Dressing, p.202
  Rye bread, p.122

* Easy Aduki Bean Soup, p. 177 or 183
  Millet Pilaf casserole, p.254-255
  Tomato Basil Salad, p.192

* Vegetable foo yung, p.228
  Salad with ginger/tahini dressing, p.203
  Oatmeal Cookies, p.283

* Creamy Black Bean Soup, p.177 or 183
  Rainbow Salad with Oil and Vinegar Dressing, p.202
  Applesauce Muffins, p.128

* Vegetable Soup, p.179 or 180
  Baked squash, with Wild Rice Stuffing, p.236
  Raw Fruit Pie, p.289

* Hot Borscht, p.179
  Vegetable Pie, p.229
  Green Salad with Watercress Dressing, p.203

* Lentil Vegetable Soup, p.177 or 183
  Sweet Potato Scallion Pie, p.235
  Watercress Endive Salad, p.193, with lemon juice + dill

* Quick potato soup, p.188
  Sandwich: rye bread, p.122; mayonnaise; sprouts
      slices of avocado and tomato; romaine lettuce.
  Carob chip cookies, p.282

* Blended salad, p.193
  Avocado/sunchoke salad, p.193
  Essene bread, p.121, with tahini or raw butter on top

* Gaspacho, p.187
  Lentil walnut burgers, p.273
  Salad with tahini-ginger dressing, p.203
  Peach ice cream, p.295

* Raw borscht, p.186
  Sunburgers, p.230
  Salad with Quick carrot dressing, p.201

* All American pizza, p.229
  Herbal ginger ale, p.165
  Salad with Oil & vinegar dressing, p.201 or 202
  Oatmeal cookies, p.283

* Lemon-Egg Soup, p.184
  Tomato-zucchini saute, p.226
  Salad with Watercress dressing, p.203
  Gingerbread, p.126

* Easy split pea soup, p.177
  Mock tabouli, p.258
  Salad with Quick ginger-soy dressing, p.201
  Fresh fruit topped with nut milk, p.156

* Italian tofu-noodles, p.265
  Watercress-endive salad, p.193
      with Ruth Duffy's dressing, p.202
  Sesame rice, p.253
  Banana ice cream, p.294

* Pecan-Noodle salad, p.266
  Broiled tofu, p.276
  Brilliant Mary, p.161
  Millet banana bread, p.124

* Quick carrot soup, p.176
  Sandwich: whole grain pita bread with miso-tahini
      spread, p.208; sunflower seeds; sliced cucumber;
      sliced onion; alfalfa sprouts, p.109
  Carob brownie, p.281

* Wild Rice and Bean Loaf with Mushroom Gravy, p.274
  Mixed Vegetable Salad with Oil and Vinegar, p.202

* Fruit dinner: Tropical Delight, p.198
      with Quick Fruit Dressing, p.201

GLOSSARY OF TERMS

AGAR AGAR (KANTEN). A gelatinous sea vegetable used like gelatin to make gelled salads and desserts. Agar comes in flake, powder or stick form.

ARROWROOT. The finely ground tuberous root of certain plants from the tropical West Indies, including the maranta (a house plant, called "prayer plant"). Arrowroot has the same uses as cornstarch; i.e. as a thickener for soups, puddings and sauces. Arrowroot is superior to cornstarch because it contains trace minerals and calcium. Cornstarch has no nutritional value, since it is processed. For the use of arrowroot in cooking, see p.208.

BRAN. The outer layer, or husk of a grain, such as wheat bran, corn bran, rye bran, oat bran, rice bran, etc. The husk is mostly fiber, the indigestible part of a food. Fiber passes into the lower bowel, or colon, absorbing water and adding bulk to the stool, thereby helping bowel regularity.

BREWERS YEAST. The micro-organism used by brewers to ferment barley and hops into beer. It is often washed off and sold as a supplement. It is 50% protein, high in B complex vitamins, chromium, selenium, and traces of iron, calcium and potassium.

BUCKWHEAT. A grain-like food used in "natural food" cooking. Botanically, it is a fruit rather than a grain, since its seeds are produced from flowers.
       Unlike grains, such as wheat or rice, which contain a bran, germ and endosperm, the buckwheat seed contains only a shell and a kernel inside the shell, called "groat". The groat is the edible portion and is used in the same way grains are used, since they have similar characteristics. For example, the groats are ground into flour and used in pancakes or made into buckwheat soba noodles. The groats are roasted (called "kasha") and eaten as a cereal or side dish, used in loaves, stuffings, etc.
       When the buckwheat sprouts, it first forms small heart shaped leaves, called buckwheat greens, tender delicacies often used in natural food preparation, especially in a raw food diet.
       Note that buckwheat is not wheat. (Those with wheat allergies can often tolerate buckwheat.) The name buckwheat derives from its Dutch name "Boekweit", meaning "beech wheat". The Dutch thought it looked like tiny beech nuts, but when the English colonists heard the name, they translated it as buckwheat.
       Buckwheat is high in B vitamins, particularly B1, B3 and B6, Vitamin A, calcium, phosphorous, iron, potassium, protein (especially the amino acid lysine), complex carbohydrate, and is a good source of rutin, a flavonoid important for capillary integrity.

CAROB. A pod found on a tree called locust honey tree, an evergreen leguminous tree. Carob is also called "St. John's Bread" since it is said that St. John fed on carob when in the wilderness. The carob pod can be eaten as is, or ground into a powder and used to give a chocolate - like taste to beverages, brownies, etc.

For real chocolate lovers, carob should not be expected to taste like chocolate. It has its own delicious flavor. It is rich in vitamins A and B complex, as well as many trace minerals, calcium, potassium, phosphorus and magnesium. It costs about the same as chocolate and, unlike chocolate, is naturally sweet, low in calories and low in fat. (Be sure to purchase it unsweetened. Sweeten it yourself with pure sweeteners.)

COLD-PRESSED. Oil is extracted from a nut, seed or bean with mechanical pressure, rather than high heats. The term "cold pressed" can literally only apply to olive or sesame oil since these are the only two nuts/seeds which yield enough oil without first being heated. Other unrefined oils have been pressed after being heated to a temperature of 200° to 250°. However, "cold pressed" oils are also produced without the use of chemicals, and are not subjected to a bleaching process. Therefore, be sure your oils say "cold pressed" on the labels. They can be purchased in health food stores.

DULSE. A red seaweed containing many trace minerals, especially iodine. Dulse can be eaten straight from the bag, or can be added to soups, grain or vegetable dishes, etc. It can be used whole or ground.

ENZYME. A protein occurring naturally throughout the body, acting as a kind of catalyst for all metabolic functions.

HYDROGENATION. A process in which a liquid oil is converted to a hard shortening for longer shelf life and for a different texture. The liquid unsaturated oil is converted to a saturated, or hard form, by chemically forcing it to accept (or saturating it with) hydrogen ions. (See "Saturated" and "Unsaturated".) The process is done with high heats and toxic chemicals, such as methyl silicone and propyl gallate. The mixture is then bleached with chemicals to whiten it to a more commercially saleable product.

KASHA. Roasted buckwheat groats. See "Buckwheat".

KEFIR MILK ("RIFEK") is a liquid, yogurt-like cultured dairy product. It is made by adding a culture, containing "friendly bacteria" - lactobacillus caucasicus, lactobacillus acidophilus and lactobacillus bulgaricus - to whole, pasteurized milk. These "friendly bacteria" are said to aid the digestive system, and help restore and maintain well-balanced intestinal flora.

Kefir cheese, made from kefir milk, has the texture and taste of a delicious, rich sour cream.

The label may read "rifek" (kefir spelled backwards) instead of kefir. The generic name "kefir" has been prohibited in New York State, since the product made in New York State does not contain the fermenting, effervescing, alcoholic characteristics of the kefir made in Europe and Asia.

KELP. A seaweed, usually ground to a powder and used as a salt substitute, since it has a salty flavor. It is high in natural iodine and trace minerals. (It will add a darker color to the foods to which it is added.)

KOMBU. A brown seaweed, used in Japanese and "natural food" cooking.

KUZU OR KUDZU. (Pronounced "koo'zoo" or "kood'zoo", except in the deep South, where it is pronounced "kud'zoo".) It is a natural root starch used as a superb thickener and jelling agent in natural food cooking. It is also said to contain fine medicinal properties. Whole books have been written on the value of kudzu.

Kudzu is a vine from the Orient, introduced to the U.S. in 1876. There it was praised in the South, as it helped prevent soil erosion, and it revitalized the soil and made an excellent forage crop. The initial praise quickly died down, however, as the fast-growing vine seemed to take over the South, engulfing telephone poles, abandoned sites, and smothering trees by blocking out the sunlight. It was joked that the way to plant kudzu was to "plant it and run".

Unfortunately, the value of the kudzu root has not been discovered in the South. It is harvested, with great expense and difficulty in the Orient and sold in Oriental and natural food stores as small white chunks packaged in clear plastic bags, usually labeled "kuzu". For the use of kudzu in cooking, see p.207.

LIVE FOODS. Unprocessed, uncooked foods in their natural, whole state, such as sprouts. Live foods still contain and impart to you the "breath of life".

**MISO**. Fermented soybean paste, or soybean plus grain paste (such as rice or barley miso). It is the dark paste that is packaged in a clear, plastic bag or in a tub container.

Miso is used in natural food cooking in soups, sauces, etc. It is extremely salty, as salt is used in the fermenting process along with koji (a starter) and water.

**NUT MILK**. A milky looking liquid made by blending nuts and seeds, or nut butters, with water. It can be used in place of milk in any recipe, is usually non-allergenic and is high in protein, vitamins and minerals. See "Beverages", pp.151 and 154-156.

**NORI**. A seaweed, used in Oriental and "natural food" cooking.

**ORGANICALLY GROWN**. Organically grown food is food grown without the use of pesticides or artificial fertilizers, and grown in soil whose humus and mineral content is increased by additions of organic matter and natural mineral fertilizers. It is food that has not been treated with preservatives, hormones, antibiotics, etc.

**REJUVELAC**. Fermented beverage drained off soaked grain, usually soft pastry wheat, which is soaked in water overnight or longer. Rejuvelac is high in vitamins E, B and K and enzymes. It is a predigested food so it may aid digestion and provide friendly bacteria for the colon. See "Beverages", pp.152 and 167.

**SATURATED FAT**. Saturated fats tend to be of animal origin, and are usually hard at room temperature. In its molecular structure, it contains a large proportion of saturated fatty acids. A fatty acid is a substance which gives fats their different flavors, textures and melting points. When a fatty acid is "saturated", it has a chemical structure which is "saturated" with hydrogen ions. That is, it cannot accept any additional hydrogen ions.

**SEA SALT**. The salt from sea water, dried naturally in the sun. It does not contain chemicals added to make it flow freely, as does refined salt. In addition, sea salt is 75% sodium chloride, containing other minerals as well as sodium. Therefore, it is more balanced then common table salt, which is pure sodium chloride.

**SHOYU**. "Soy Sauce". The liquid that results from fermenting soybeans, roasted cracked wheat, salt and well water.

**SPROUT**. The shoot of a plant, such as alfalfa, mung, lentil, etc. It is high in enzymes, vitamins, minerals, protein and life force. See "Sprouts", p.107.

TAHINI. Sesame seed paste, or sesame seed butter, made by grinding sesame seeds. It is something like peanut butter, but is made with sesame seeds instead of peanuts. (Peanut butter is more difficult to digest, and is often contaminated with a mold which has been found to be cancer-causing.)

Use tahini as a spread on bread or crackers, make a sauce, dip or dressing with it. Blend it with water and honey for a drink. Add it to oatmeal or other grains. Put it in candies or desserts. It's delicious.

TAMARI. "Soy Sauce". Originally the liquid that resulted from fermenting soybeans, salt and koji (a mold starter). Sometimes it has wheat added, to alter the flavor.

TEMPEH. Fermented cooked soy beans. It is made by adding a rhizopus culture to lightly cooked soybeans, and letting them stand in a warm place overnight. The culture partially digests the beans, and binds them together with a fine, white mycelium.

TOFU. Soybean curd, first made in China over 2,000 years ago and used as a primary source of protein in the East Asian diet.

Tofu is the white block you may see sitting in water in oriental or vegetable markets. It also comes in a package, refrigerated in health food stores. The packaged tofu is better, because it is less likely to be contaminated from sitting out in the open. However, make sure it contains no toxic additives. (See pp.302-305 for a list of toxic additives.)

To make Tofu, soybeans are soaked overnight, ground into a puree and cooked in steam. The soy milk is squeezed from the pulp, and Nigari (seawater extract) is added as a solidifier. The milk separates into curd and whey. The whey is ladled off and the curd is put into a tray lined with cheesecloth and then pressed with weights.

Tofu is used in "natural food" cooking as a source of protein. It is a great base for dips, ice creams, pies, blender drinks, etc. Entire books have been written on the uses of tofu. The simplest way to begin using it is to cut it in chunks and add it to soups.

TRITICALE. A hybrid grain, resulting from crossing wheat and rye seeds. It has 16.4% more protein than most of the cereal grains. Although it is a cross-breed, it can reproduce itself. Because of its high amino acid balance, it has a biological value close to that of eggs and meat -- closer than rye or wheat by themselves.

UMEBOSHI. Plums pickled in brine. Unripe apricots, or "plums" are sprinkled with salt, arranged in layers in wooden kegs, earthenware crocks, or concrete vats lined with fiberglass. Then they are compressed by a layer of straw mats, a wooden lid and large stones. For 1-2 months the pickling process is carried out by salt and some fermentation enzymes which cause the production of lactic acid, one of the most important components of umeboshi, together with citric acid.

UNSATURATED FAT. A fat which is so constituted chemically that it is able to accept additional hydrogen ions. That is, it is not "saturated" with hydrogen ions. (See "Saturated Fats".) Unsaturated fatty acids are usually liquid at room temperature, and are primarily derived from vegetables, nuts or seeds, such as sunflower or sesame oil. It is thought that unsaturated fats are less likely to contribute fatty deposits in blood vessels than saturated fats.

UNSULFURED. The toxic chemical, sulfur dioxide has not been used in the processing of a food that is unsulfured. In the case of dried fruit, sulfur dioxide is often used to enhance and preserve color. The cut fruit is exposed to fumes of burning sulfur, which penetrates the fruit and inactivates the enzymes, preserving the color. (For example, sulfured dried apricots are bright orange, whereas unsulfured dried apricots are usually brown.) Sulfur fumes combine with water in the dried fruit, forming sulfurous acid, which remains in the fruit and is toxic to humans.

WAKAME. A seaweed, or sea vegetable, used in Oriental and "natural food" cooking.

WHEATGRASS. Grass grown from the wheat berry. High in enzymes, vitamins, minerals and chlorophyll. The grass is chewed, or juiced with a special juicer.

******** COOKBOOKS ********

## GENERAL

Albright, Nancy, NATURALLY GREAT FOODS. Rodale Press, Emmaus, Pennsylvania 18049.

Albright, Nancy, THE RODALE COOKBOOK. Rodale Press, Emmaus, Pennsylvania 18049.

Bricklin, Mark and Claessens, Sharon, THE NATURAL HEALING COOKBOOK, Rodale Press, Emmaus, Pennsylvania.

Graf, Eva, and Seagrave, Mitch, THE GOOD BOOK COOKBOOK - Transition Recipes from The Center of The Light. The Church of Christ Consciousness, New Marlboro, Massachusetts.

Hurd, Frank J. and Rosalie, TEN TALENTS. College Press, Chisholm, Minnesota.

Jensen, Dr. Bernard, BLENDING MAGIC. Bernard Jensen Products, P.O. Box 8, Solana Beach, California 92075.

Kenda, Margaret Elizabeth & Williams, Phyllis S., THE NATURAL BABY FOOD COOKBOOK. Avon Books, The Hearst Corporation. 959 8th Avenue, New York, New York.

Kinderlehrer, Jane, CONFESSIONS OF A SNEAKY ORGANIC COOK. New American Library. P.O. Box 999, Bergenfield, New Jersey, 07621. (Out of Print.)

Rombauer, Irma S. & Becker, Marion Rombauer, JOY OF COOKING. The Bobbs & Merrill Co., Inc., Howard W. Sams & Co., Inc. 4300 West 62nd Street, Indianapolis, Indiana. Note: This is a wonderful basic cookbook, but has lots of sugar. Use your conversion hints.

Walker, Dr. N.W., DIET AND SALAD. Norwalk Press, Publishers. 2218 East Magnolia, Phoenix, Arizona 85034.

## VEGETARIAN

Colbin, Annemarie, THE BOOK OF WHOLE MEALS. Autumn Press, Inc., 25 Dwight St., Brookline, Massachusetts 02146.

Ford, Marjorie Winn; Hillyard, Susan; Koock, Mary Faulk, THE DEAF SMITH COUNTRY COOKBOOK. Collier Books, Macmillan Publishing Co., 866 Third Avenue, New York, New York 10022.

Katzen, Mollie, MOOSEWOOD COOKBOOK. Ten Speed Press. P.O. Box 7123. Berkeley, California 94707.

Robertson, Laurel, LAUREL'S KITCHEN, Carol Flinders and Bronwen Godfrey, Bantam Books.

Shurtleff, William and Aoyagi, Akiko, THE BOOK OF KUDZU, Autumn Press, 7 Littell Road, Brookline, Mass.02146.


## FOR RAW FOODS

Acciardo, Marcia, LIGHT EATING FOR SURVIVAL. Omando D'Press. P.O. Box 255, Wethersfield, Connecticut, 06109.

Bragg, Dr. Paul, SALT-FREE SAUERKRAUT.

Kulvinskas, Victoras, LOVE YOUR BODY. Omando D'Press. P.O. Box 255, Wethersfield, Connecticut, 06109.

Wigmore, Dr. Ann, RECIPES FOR LIFE. Rising Sun Publications, 25 Exeter Street, Boston, Massachusetts 02116.


## SUGAR-FREE DESSERTS

Dworkin, Stan and Floss, GOOD GOODIES. Rodale Press, Emmaus, Pennsylvania 18049.

Martin, Faye, NATURALLY DELICIOUS DESSERTS & SNACKS. Rodale Press, Emmaus, Pennsylvania 18049.


******** GENERAL REFERENCE ********

Adams, Ruth and Murray, Frank, BODY, MIND AND THE B VITAMINS, Larchmont Books.

Cheraskin, E., M.D., D.M.D., and Ringsdorf, William Jr., D.M.D. M.S., NEW HOPE FOR INCURABLE DISEASES, Exposition Press, Inc., 50 Jerico Turnpike, Jerico, New York 11753.

Coca, Arthur F., M.D., THE PULSE TEST, Lyle Stuart, 225 Lafayette Street, New York, New York, 10012.

Consolidated Book Publishers for Educational Book Club, Inc., WEBSTER ENCYCLOPEDIC DICTIONARY, 1968.

Donsbach, Kurt W., Ph.D., BASIC NUTRITION FACTS, The International Institute of Natural Health Sciences, Huntington Beach, California.

Donsbach, Kurt W. and Nittler, Alan H., M.D., "HEART ATTACK", The International Institute of National Health Sciences, P.O. Box 5550, Huntington Beach, California 92646.

Feingold, Ben F., M.D., WHY YOUR CHILD IS HYPERACTIVE, Random House.

Garten, Max, N.D., D.C., "CIVILIZED" DISEASES AND THEIR CIRCUMVENTION, Maxmillian World Publishers, Inc., San Jose, California 95152.

Gerson, Max, M.D., A CANCER THERAPY, RESULTS OF FIFTY CASES, Totality Books, P.O. Box 1035, Del Mar, California 92014.

Goldbeck, Nikki and David, THE SUPERMARKET HANDBOOK, Signet Books, The New American Library, Inc., 1301 Avenue of the Americas, New York, New York 10019.

Goodhart, Robert F., M.D., D.M.S., and Shils, Maurice E., M.D., Sc.D., MODERN NUTRITION IN HEALTH AND DISEASE, Sixth Edition, Lea and Febiger, Philadelphia, Pennsylvania.

Houben, Milton and Kropf, William, M.D., HARMFUL FOOD ADDITIVES, Ashley Books, Inc., Port Washington, New York 11050.

Hunter, Beatrice Trum, BEATRICE TRUM HUNTER'S ADDITIVES BOOK, Keats Publishing, Inc., 36 Grove Street, New Canaan, Conn. 06840.

Hunter, Beatrice Trum, CONSUMER BEWARE, A Touchstone Book, Simon and Schuster, Rockefeller Center, 1230 Avenue of the Americas, New York, New York 10020.

Jackson, Dr. Michael; Liebman, Bonnie F., and Moyer, Greg, SALT: THE BRAND NAME GUIDE TO SODIUM CONTENT, Workman Publishing Co., New York, New York.

Jarvis, D.C., M.D., FOLK MEDICINE, A Fawcett Crest Book, Fawcett Publications, Inc., Greenwich, Connecticut.

Jensen, Bernard, D.C., DOCTOR PATIENT HANDBOOK, Bernard Jensen Enterprises, Route 1, Box 52, Escondido, California, 92025.

Jones, Susan Smith, THE MAIN INGREDIENTS: POSITIVE THINKING, EXERCISE AND DIET, Biworld Publishers, Provo, Utah.

Kulvinskas, Viktoras ,M.S., N.D., NUTRITIONAL EVALUATION OF SPROUTS AND GRASSES, O'Mango Press, P.O. Box 255, Wethersfield, Connecticut 06109.

Lappe, Frances Moore, DIET FOR A SMALL PLANET, Ballantine Books, A Division of Random House, Inc., 201 East 50th Street, New York, New York 10022.

Longgood, William, THE POISONS IN YOUR FOOD, Pyramid Publications, New York, New York.

National Academy of Sciences, Washington, D.C., RECOMMENDED DIETARY ALLOWANCES. Ninth Revised Edition, 1980. Office of Publications, National Academy of Sciences, 2101 Constitution Avenue N.W., Washington, D.C., 20418.

Null, Gary, THE NEW VEGETARIAN, William Morrow and Company, Inc., 105 Madison Avenue, New York, New York 10016.

The Nutrition Foundation, Inc., PRESENT KNOWLEDGE IN NUTRITION, Fourth Edition, 888 Seventeenth Street N.W., Washington, D.C.

Nutrition Publications, Inc., MANUAL OF CLINICAL NUTRITION, Pleasantville, New Jersey.

Nutrition Search, Inc., NUTRITION ALMANAC, McGraw Hill Book Company.

Passwater, Richard A., SUPER NUTRITION, Pocket Books, 1230 Avenue of the Americas, New York 10020.

Pinkham, Mary Ellen and Higginbotham, Pearl, MARY ELLEN'S BEST OF HELPFUL HINTS. Warner Books, Inc., 75 Rockefeller Plaza, New York, New York 10019.

Riker, Tom and Roberts, Richard, THE DIRECTORY OF NATURAL AND HEALTH FOODS. Paragon Books, G.P. Putnam's Sons, 200 Madison Avenue , New York, New York 10016.

Rodale, J.I. and Staff, COMPLETE BOOK OF FOOD AND NUTRITION, Emmaus, Pennsylvania.

Ruben, David, M.D., THE SAVE YOUR LIFE DIET, Random House.

Schauss, Alexander, DIET, CRIME AND DELINQUENCY, Parker House, 2340 Parker Street, Berkeley, California, 94704.

U.S. Department of Agriculture, HANDBOOK OF THE NUTRITIONAL CONTENT OF FOODS, Dover Publications, Inc., New York, New York.

Williams, Roger J., NUTRITION AGAINST DISEASE, International Institute of Natural Health Sciences, Inc., P.O. Box 5550, Huntington Beach, California 92646.

The Williams and Wilkins Co., STEDMAN'S MEDICAL DICTIONARY, 23rd Edition, Baltimore, Maryland.

Whittlesey, Marietta, KILLER SALT, Avon Books, The Hearst Corp., 959 5th Avenue, New York, New York, 10019.


### ARTICLES

Bland, Jeffrey, Ph.D., and Berquist, Barbara, "NUTRIENT CONTENT OF GERMINATED SEEDS", Journal of the John Bastyr College of Naturopathic Medicine, Vol. 2; No. 1, June, 1980, pp. 3-8.

DiSogra, Charles, M.P.H. and Groll, Lorelei, Ed.D., R.D. "NUTRITION AND CANCER PREVENTION: A GUIDE TO FOOD CHOICES", A booklet supported by a Cancer Control Grant from The American Cancer Society.

Flatto, Edwin, M.D. "THE MERITS OF HONEY", A reprint in the "Cancer Forum" from an article in "Herald of Health" magazine.

Furman, Arthur F., D.D.S., "ALUMINUM & ALZHEIMER'S DISEASE", "Let's Live", May, 1981, pp.65-68.

Med. Counterpoint, 6 (Nov.):39."BOVINE MILK XANTHINE OXIDASE AS ONE OF THE DIETARY CAUSES OF EARLY ATHEROCLEROSIS".

Meyerowitz, Steve (Sproutman), "INSTRUCTIONS FOR THE FLAXSEED SPROUT BAG", The Sprout House, 210 Riverside Drive, New York, NY 10025.

Meyerowitz, Steve, (Sproutman), "INSTRUCTIONS FOR THE ORIGINAL BASKET SPROUTER", The Sprout House, 210 Riverside Drive, New York, New York 10025.

Meyerowitz, Steve "A NEW WAY OF SPROUTING", "Prevention", March 1983, Vol. 35, No.3, p. 98.

"NUTRITION REVIEWS", Vol. 33, #4, April 1975, pp.123-125.

Oster, Kurt A., "PLASMALOGEN DISEASES: A NEW CONCEPT OF THE ETIOLOGY OF THE ATHEROSCLEROTIC PROCESS", "American Journal of Clinical Research, 1971. 2:30.

Oster, Kurt A., "PLASMALOGENS", "New England Journal of Medicine, 1974, 290:913.

"Prevention" Magazine, "A HEALTH FOOD DICTIONARY", Sept.'78-Jan.'81, Emmaus, Pennsylvania.

Shore, David, M.D. and Wyatt, Richard Jed, M.D., "ALUMINUM AND ALZHEIMER"S DISEASE", The Journal of Nervous and Mental Disease, Vol:171, #9, pp.553-558.

******** FOOTNOTES ********

Section I, Chapter 1, Food Cravings, pp.30-32.
  #1. Diet, Crime and Delinquency, p.81.
Section II, Chapter 1, Choosing Foods for Health,pp.35-46.
  Whole Grains, p.36.
      #1. Nutrition Almanac, p.88;  Handbook of the Nutri-
          tional Content of Foods - Grains in Tables 1 &
          2,  pp. 6-121.
      #2. The New Vegetarian, p.66.
      #3. The Save Your Life Diet, pp.89-105.
      #4. Nutrition Almanac, p.187; Diet for a Small
          Planet, pp.95-118.
      #5. "Civilized" Diseases, p.198.
  Sprouts, p.37.
      #1. Recipes for Life, p.12;  Nutritional Evaluation
          of Sprouts and Grasses
  Beans and Peas, p.37.
      #1. Nutrition Almanac, P.188.
      #2. Recipes for Life, p.12; Nutritional Evaluation
          of Sprouts and Grasses
      #3. Diet for a Small Planet, pp.95-98.
  Nuts and Seeds, p.38.
      #1. Mental and Elemental Nutrients, p.416; The Pulse
          Test, pp.9-11, 33-50.
      #2. Diet and Disease, pp.211-212;  Modern Nutrition
          in Health and Disease, p.518.
      #3. Nutrition Almanac, p. 191.
      #4.
  Eggs, pp.38-39.
      #1. Nutrition Almanac, p.186; Mental and Elemental
          Nutrients, p.83.
      #2. Diet and Disease, pp.22-23, Protein destruction
          through heating.
      #3. Nutrition Almanac, p. 186
      #4. New Vegetarian, p.123; Consumer Beware, pp.166-
          179.
      #5. Nutrition Almanac, p.186; Nutrition Against Dis-
          ease, p.74.
      #6. Nutrition Against Disease, p.232; Mental and
          Elemental Nutrients, pp.82, 84-87;  Save Your
          Life Diet, p.45-47.
  Fish, p.39.
      #1. Nutrition Almanac, p.186.
      #2. New Vegetarian, p.51;  Modern Nutrition in
          Health and Disease, p.484.
  Meat, p.40.
      #1. Nutrition Almanac, p.186.
      #2. New Vegetarian, pp.115-118, 76-86; Consumer
          Beware, pp. 111-166.
  Dairy, p.40.
      #1. New Vegetarian, p.56; "Civilized" Diseases,
          pp.75-76
      #2. Nutrition Against Disease, p.182; New
          Vegetarian, p.98.

Oils, p.41.
    #1. Modern Nutrition in Health and Disease, p.504;
      Mental and Elemental Nutrients, p.25; Present
      Knowledge in Nutrition, pp.102 and 313.
    #2. Modern Nutrition in Health and Disease, p.475.
Fruits, p.42.
    #1. Nutrition Almanac, p.186
Vegetables, p.42.
    #1. Nutrition Almanac, p.193.
    #2. Nutrition Almanac, p.195.
Sweeteners, p.43.
    #1. Folk Medicine, pp.100-102; "The Merits of
      Honey".

Section II, Chapter 2, Avoiding Stressful Foods, pp.47-55.
    Introduction, p.48.
      #1. "Good Morning America" Health Test,2/21/84. Pre-
      pared in cooperation with the National Centers
      for Disease Control, U.S. Dept. of Health and
      Human Services.
    Sugar, p.49.
      #1. "Civilized" Diseases, p.31.
      #2. Susceptibility to disease: Super Nutrition,
      p.145; Sweet and Dangerous, p.164-165; New Hope
      for Incurable Disease, pp.163-165;
      Tooth decay and gum disease: Nutrition Against
      Disease, p.119; Super Nutrition, p.145; Present
      Knowledge in Nutrition, pp.488-504; Sweet and
      Dangerous, p.132; New Vegetarian, pp.269-271.
      Acne: Sweet and Dangerous, pp.84-86.
      Obesity: Nutrition Against Disease, p.169; Super
      Nutrition, p.145; New Vegetarian, p.274; New
      Hope for Incurable Disease, p.157; Present
      Knowledge in Nutrition, p.37.
      Hypoglycemia: Super Nutrition, p.145; Diet and
      Disease, p.55; Sweet and Dangerous, pp.118-121.
      Diabetes: New Vegetarian, p.274; Present Know-
      ledge in Nutrition, p.35; New Hope for Incurable
      Diseases, p.165; "Civilized" Diseases, pp.26,
      28 and 33.
      Arthritis: "Civilized" Diseases, p.26; Sweet and
      Dangerous, pp.138-139.
      Heart Disease: Nutrition Against Disease, p.85;
      Present Knowledge in Nutrition, p.35; Super
      Nutrition, pp.142-143; New Vegetarian, p.274;
      Diet and Disease, pp.259,265,334; Modern
      Nutrition in Health and Disease, pp.1048 and
      798.
      Alcoholism: Super Nutrition, p.145; New Hope
      for Incurable Disease, pp.58,59,62.
      Drug Addiction: Diet, Crime and Delinquency,
      pp.24-25.
      Schizophrenia: Super Nutrition, p.145.

Section II, Chapter 2, cont.
   Sugar, cont.
         Nervous Disorders: Killer Salt, p.43; Super
         Nutrition, p.145.
         Behavior Problems: Diet, Crime and Delinquency,
         pp.24-25.
         Poor digestion and assimilation: New Vegetarian,
         p.201; Super Nutrition, p.145.
   Salt, p.50.
      #3. Water balance in cells: Killer Salt, p.78;
         Cancer Therapy, pp.153-166; Food is Your Best
         Medicine, p.221.
         Circulatory system: Food is Your Best Medicine,
         p.223.
         Potassium deficiency: Cancer Therapy, pp.153-
         166.
         Digestive disorders: Basic Nutrition Facts,
         p.16.
         Kidney disease: Food is Your Best Medicine,
         p.221; Killer Salt, pp.54 and 66; Modern Nutri-
         tion in Health and Disease, p.1019.
         Nervous disorders: Killer Salt, pp.42-45,52.
         Hypertension: Modern Nutrition in Health and
         Disease, pp. 1019, 1008; Killer Salt, pp.61 and
         101.
         Heart disease: Food is Your Best Medicine,
         p.223; Nutrition Against Disease, p.86; Modern
         Nutrition in Health and Disease, p.1019.
         Cancer: Cancer Therapy, pp.153-166; Diet and
         Disease, pp.214-216,228; "Civilized" Diseases,
         p.255.
   Additives, p.50.
      #1. Schizophrenia: Mental and Elemental Nutrients,
         p.412.
         Hyperactivity: Why Your Child is Hyperactive,
         Chapter 7; Diet, Crime and Delinquency, pp.50-53
         Cancer: Nutrition and Cancer, p.13
      #2. Harmful Food Additives, pp.65 and 19-26.
   Processed and Refined Flour, Grains, Cereals and
   Noodles, p.51.
      #1. Modern Nutrition in Health and Disease, pp.498-
         499.
      #2. Mental and Elemental Nutrients, New Hope for
         Incurable Disease, p.157.
      #3. Nutrition Against Disease, pp.79 and 201-205.
      #4. New Vegetarian, p.267.
      #5. Susceptibility to disease: New Hope for Incura-
         ble Disease, p.163.
         Obesity: New Vegetarian, pp.269-271; Save Your
         Life Diet, pp.102-105; Present Knowledge in
         Nutrition, Chapter 5.

Processed and Refined Grains, cont.
>Digestion, metabolism and elimination: Present Knowledge in Nutrition, Chapter 38; New Vegetarian, pp.70-77; Save Your Life Diet.
>Ulcers and urinary tract infections: New Vegetarian, pp.269-271.
>Nutrient deficiencies: Modern Nutrition in Health and Disease, pp.498-499; New Hope for Incurable Disease, p.157 & 163.
>Nervous disorders, schizophrenia, hyperactivity: Mental and Elemental Nutrients, p.412.
>Cancer: Present Knowledge in Nutrition, chapter 38; New Vegetarian, pp.269-271; Save Your Life Diet, pp.29-35,45 & 46.
>Hemmorhoids and Varicose veins: Save Your Life Diet; New Vegetarian, pp.269-271;
>Heart Disease: Present Knowledge In Nutrition, Chapter 5 & p.35; Diet & Disease, p.334; New Vegetarian, pp.269-271; Save Your Life Diet, pp.45-48.
>Diabetes: New Vegetarian, pp.269-271; Present Knowledge in Nutrition, p.358.

Meats, p.52.
>#1. Consumer Beware, pp.148-162.
>#2. New Vegetarian, pp.115-118;72-74;76-77;82-86.

Oils, pp.53-54.
>#1. Modern Nutrition in Health and Disease, p.120.
>#2. New Vegetarian, pp.242,250-252; Nutrition Against Disease, p.245; Present Knowledge in Nutrition, p.37.
>#3. Nutrition and Cancer Prevention, p.23.
>#4. Modern Nutrition in Health and Disease, p.504; Mental and Elemental Nutrients, p.25; Present Knowledge in Nutrition, pp.313 & 102.
>#5. Common Food Additives,p.56; Nutrition Against Disease, p.245; Modern Nutrition in Health and Disease, p.503.
>#6. New Vegetarian, pp.245,255; Modern Nutrition in Health and Disease, p.503; Present Knowledge in Nutrition, p.37; New Vegetarian, pp.250-252.
>#7. Common Food Additives, p.56.

Alcohol, p.54.
>#1. Diet, Crime and Delinquency, pp.65-66; New Hope for Incurable Diseases, p.62; Nutrition Against Disease, pp.169-170.

Milk, p.55.
>#1. Diet, Crime and Delinquency, pp.13-14; Don't Drink Your Milk,pp.10-15,17,23,53; Milk Intolerances and Rejection, pp.1,4,12-13; Nutrition Against Disease, pp.188,192; Food is Your Best Medicine, p.164; Mental & Elemental Nutrients, pp.416,417.
>#2. Don't Drink Your Milk, pp.32-33; Basic Nutrition Facts, p.22.

Milk, cont.
>    Heating proteins: New Vegetarian, p.50; Diet and Disease, p.22.
>    Tests done on homogenization by Dr. Kurt Oster: "Civilized" Diseases, p.75; The Main Ingredients, p.13; Articles by Kurt Oster in American Journal of Clinical Research, New England Journal of Medicine and Med. Counterpoint. (See Bibliography, "Articles".).
>    #3. Modern Nutrition in Health and Disease,pp.470, 491; New Vegetarian, pp.89-92.

Caffeine, p.55.
>    #1. Ulcers: tests done by Dr. Edward Judd of University of Minnesota, and Roth & Ivy of Northwestern University School of Medicine. Basic Nutrition Facts, p.29; "Civilized" Diseases, p.79.
>    #2. Basic Nutrition Facts, p.29.
>    #3. Intestinal disorders: Modern Nutrition in Health and Disease, pp.35-37.
>    #4. Nutrition Almanac, p.194.; "Civilized" Diseases, p.78.

Tannin, p.54.
>    #5. Basic Nutrition Facts, p.29; Harmful Food Additives, p.26.

Chocolate, p.54.
>    #1. Naturally Great Foods, p.295.
>    #2. Basic Nutrition Facts, p.29;
>    #3. Rodale Cookbook, p.366; Complete Book of Food and Nutrition, p.452; Modern Nutrition in Health and Disease, p.476.
>    #4. Tests done with allergies to chocolate by Dr. Joseph A. Fries, Director of the Allergy Service at the Methodist Hospital of Brooklyn, Annals of Allergy, Sept, 66. 70% of allergy-prone children reacted to chocolate: Naturally Great Foods, pp.295-296; Mental and Elemental Nutrients, p.416 ; Food is Your Best Medicine, p.164; Hearing Before the Select Committee on Nutrition, Volume 2, pp.27-29; Modern Nutrition in Health and Disease, p.475; Diet,Crime and Delinquency, pp.80-81.

Allergens, p.56.
>    #1. Diet, Crime and Delinquency, pp.75-79,81; Food is Your Best Medicine, p.164; Mental and Elemental Nutrients, p.415; Modern Nutrition in Health and Disease, p.475; Hearing Before the Select Committee on Nutrition, Volume 2, pp.27-29.
>    #2. Diet, Crime and Delinquency, p.81.
>    #3. Food is Your Best Medicine, p.164; Mental and Elemental Nutrients, p.416; Pulse Test, pp. 9-11 33-50.

Section 11, Chapter 5
    Equipment & Utensils, p.69.
        #1. Aluminum: "Aluminum and Alzheimer's Disease",
            Arthur F. Furman, D.D.S.; "Aluminum and Alzhei-
            mer's Disease, David Shore, M.D. and Richard Jed
            Wyatt, M.D.
    Chapter 8 - Protein in a Vegetarian Diet, p.87.
        #1. Diet for a Small Planet pp.95-118.
    Chapter 10 - Basic Food Preparation
    Preparing Foods to Preserve Nutrients, p.98.
        #1. Diet and Disease, p.21; New Hope for Incurable
            Disease, p.27.
        #2. Nutrition Reviews,Vol.33,#4,April,'75,
            pp.123-125; Civilized Diseases, pp.194-195; Diet
            and Disease, pp.21-23; New Vegetarian, p.50;
            Modern Nutrition in Health and Disease,
            pp.475-498.
        #3. Civilized Diseases, p.194; New Vegetarian, pp.
            250-252; Nutrition Against Disease, p.245.
        #4. Modern Nutrition in Health and Disease, p.120.
Section 111, Recipes
    Sprouts, pp.108-109.
        #1. Recipes for Life, p.12; Nutritional Evaluation
            of Sprouts and Grasses; "Nutrient Content of
            Germinated Seeds".
        #2. For instructions on the "basket" and "bag"
            methods of sprouting: "Instructions for the
            Flaxseed Sprout Bag" and "Instructions for the
            Original Basket Sprouter" by Sproutman.
    Eggs, p.146.
        #1. Protein destruction through heating, Diet and
            Disease, pp.22-23.
    Beverages, p.153.
        #1. Wheatgrass information sources: Hippocrates
            Health Institute, 25 Exeter Street, Boston,
            Mass. 02116; The Sprout House, 210 Riverside
            Drive, New York, N.Y. 10025; Viktoras Kulvinskas
            P.O. Box 255, Wethersfield, Conn. 06109.
    Chicken, p.214.
        #1. New Vegetarian, pp.115-118;76-86; Consumer
            Beware, pp.148-162
    Fish, p.218.
        #1. Consumer Beware, p.180; Modern Nutrition in
            Health and Disease, p.484
    Vegetables, p.223.
        #1. Nutrition Reviews, Vol.33,#4,April'75,
            pp.123-125; Modern Nutrition in Health and Dis-
            ease, pp.497-500; Food is YOur Best Medicine, p.
            207; Diet and Disease, p.21.
Section 1V, Appendix
    Natural Food Kitchen Hints & Hints for Easy Cleaning of
    Utensils, pp.209-301.: Friends, clients, personal
    experience,"Joy of Cooking", "Mary Ellen's Best of
    Helpful Hints".

Appendix, cont.

Common Food Additives, pp.302-305: Consumer Beware, Harmful Food Additives, The Poisons in Your Food; Beatrice Trum Hunter's Additives Book; The Directory of Natural & Health Foods; The New Vegetarian; Diet,Crime and Delinquency; Why Your Child is Hyperactive; The Supermarket Handbook; Nutrition and Cancer Prevention.

Hidden Sugars, p.306: New Hope for Incurable Diseases, pp.165-169;Consumer Beware,pp.202;304-307;313-317; Laurel's Kitchen, p.405; Harmful Food Additives, pp.42,43, 50; The Natural Healing Cookbook.

Hidden Salt, p.307: Consumer Reports, March, '79; Nutrition Action, March, '78; "Salt: The Brand Name Guide to Sodium Content"; American Heart Association; "Approximate Sodium Content of Common Foods"; Consumer Beware, pp.317, 283-284.

Glossary, pp.316-321: Naturally Great Foods; The Rodale Cookbook; The Book of Kudzu; The Book of Whole Meals; Recipes for Life; Good Goodies, Naturally Delicious Desserts and Snacks; Basic Nutrition Facts; Complete Book of Food and Nutrition; The Directory of Natural and Health Foods; Nutrition Almanac; Stedman's Medical Dictionary; Webster Encyclopedic Dictionary; A Health Food Dictionary - Prevention Magazine.

SPECIAL INDEX

# CHARTS, SPECIAL LISTS & ILLUSTRATIONS CONTAINED IN THIS BOOK

SNACKS TO GO - FOR WORK OR TRAVEL
(HFS: Purchase at Health Food Store). Also refer to
Section I, Foods to Go, p.24.

BREADS & CRACKERS:
    Rice cakes or Rye crackers, HFS.
    Whole grain bread, p.122, or HFS.
    2-slice bread, p.123.
    Essene Bread or Essene rolls, HFS or see p.121.
    Corn muffins, p.127.
    Sweet Breads or muffins, pp.124-128.

BREAD SPREADS AND TOPPINGS:
    Miso Tahini Spread, pp.208-209.
    Raw butter, Almond Butter, Tahini, HFS.
    Humus, p.272.

SALADS:
    Noodle Salad, pp.275,265.       Sauerkraut, pp.196-197.
    Cranberry Relish, p.212.        Watercress Endive,p.193.
    Marinated Vegetables, p.195     Carrot Salad, p.191.
    Delicious Mixture, p.256.       Fruit Salad, p.198.
    Grain Salad, pp.257-260.        Raw Vegetables, p.194.
    Avocado & Watercress with Tofu and Sunchokes, p.192.
    1/2 Avocado, with lemon juice and soy sauce.
    Vegetable, Chicken, or Bean Salad, pp.191,275.

PORTABLE DIPS:
    Dips, pp.205-206.
    On Raw Vegetables, use Almond Butter or Tahini, HFS.
      or Miso-Tahini Spread, pp.208-209.

LOAVES AND BURGERS:
    Sunburgers, pp.230-231.    Lentil Walnut Burgers, p.273.
    Rice Cheese Nut Loaf, p.253.
    Tofu or Tempeh Burgers, HFS.

MISCELLANEOUS SNACKS:
    Dulse Seaweed, eat from package. HFS.
    Tofu plus vegetable powder and soy sauce, HFS.
    Thermos Cooked Grain, p.137.
    Leafy Greens, list on page 45 and 160.
    Sprouts, HFS or pp. 113-115.
    Nuts and Seeds Mix, pp.278,279.
    Fresh Fruits, listed on page 46.
    Sardines or Cooked Chicken.

LIQUIDS:
    Grain water, p.152.        Brilliant Mary, p.161.
    Mulled Cider, p.164.       Cranberry Juice, p.164.
    Honigar (Cider Vinegar + Honey),p.170.
    Spring Water (Hot and/or Cold), Herb Tea Bags, Pure
       Bottled Vegetable or Fruit Juices,Vegetable Bouillon
       or Miso Soup Cubes or Powder, Grain Coffee, such as
       Pero or Cafix, HFS.
    Homemade Soups, See list of "Quick Soups", p.338.

RECIPES FOR
QUICK & GOOD FOODS

PREPARATION
& COOK TIME                    RECIPE

BREADS:
30 min.      2-Slice Buckwheat Bread, p.123.

CEREALS:
10-15 min.   Oatmeal, p.133; Buckwheat Porridge, p.134;
             Cream of Grain Cereal, pp.134-135.
30 min.      Millet, pp.134,135.
5-15 min. with pre-preparation: Thermos Cereal, p.137;
             Super Cereal, p.138; Granola, p.140; Sprouted
             Cereal, p.137.

EGGS:
10-15 min.   Soft boiled, poached or fried eggs, p.146.

BEVERAGES:
5 min.       Nut milk, p.154; Soft drinks, p.165;
             Honigar (Apple Cider Vinegar & Honey), p.170
10 min.      Smoothies, pp.158-159; Green Drink,p.162.
             Vegetable juices, pp. 160-161.
20 min.      Herb teas, pp.168-169.
30 min.      Mulled juice, p.164.

SOUPS:
10 min.      Creamy Grain or Bean Soup, pp.177,183;
             Blended Left Overs, pp.176,186;
15 min.      Raw Vegetable, pp.175,187; Raw spinach, p.185.
             Raw Borscht, p.186.
15-20 min.   All soups under Create-A-Soup, p.179; Chicken
             or Fish Noodle, p.181; Creamy Root Vegetable,
             pp.185-188; Gaspacho, p.187.

SALADS:
15 min.      Avocado Watercress, p.192; Avocado Sunchoke,
             p.193; Tomato Basil, p.192; Fruit Salad, p.198
             Grain Salad, p.257;
15-20 min.   Salad on the Go, p.191; Carrot Salad, p.191;
             Blended Salad, p.193; Raw Vegetable Snacks,
             p. 194; Pea Salad, p.194.

DRESSING, DIPS & SAUCES:
5-10 min.    Quick Dressings, p.201; Quick Sauces, p.208;
             Miso-Tahini Spread, p.209.
15-20 min.   All Dressings, pp. 199-211. To make these into
             "Quick Dressings and Dips", pre-prepare them.

CHICKEN:
15-20 min.   with preparation, add Chicken to soups, salads
             casseroles, etc. See p.179, p.227, p.191.

PREPARATION
& COOK TIME          RECIPE

FISH:
10 min.      Quick Fish, p.219.
20 min.      Broiled Fish, p.220; Fish included in recipes
             pp.179 and 227.

VEGETABLES:
15-20 min.   Steamed Vegetables, p.224; Sauteed Vegetables,
             p. 225; Vegetables in Recipes, p.227; Pizza,
             p.229; Broccoli & Garlic, p.239;
For Quick left overs, pre-prepare: Sunburgers, p.230;
             Quiche, p.232; Fermeneted Seed Loaf, p.234;
             Sweet Potato Pie, p.235; Vegetable Pie, p.229.

GRAINS:
10-15 min.   Rolled Oats, p.133, Buckwheat, p.134; Bulgar,
             p.251.
30 min.      Millet, pp.134,135,251,252.
For Quick left overs, prepare grains ahead. Make cereals,
             grain water; add to soups, sauteed or steamed
             foods, salads, casseroles. See recipes,
             Create-A-Meal, p.227; Sesame rice, p.260;
             Lemon Rice Soup, p.184; Wild Rice Salad, p.257
             Creamy Grain Cereal, pp.134,135; Grain Water,
             p.166.

NOODLES:
10-15 min.   Noodles take only about 8 minutes to cook. Top
             them with a quick sauce, or add them to other
             quick recipes. Refer to Index - Noodles for
             recipe ideas, and pp.179 and 227.

BEANS:
Prepare beans ahead. Then add to casseroles, salads,
             soups, sauteed or steamed foods, etc. For
             example, Creamy Bean Soup, pp.177,183;
             Bean Salad, p.275; Quick Lentil Sauce, p.208.

TOFU:
10-15 min.   Add to quick soups, salads, etc, such as
             miso soup, p.179,182; avocado watercress
             salad, p.192.
20-25 min.   Scrambled Tofu, p.276; Broiled Tofu, p.276.

SNACKS & DESSERTS:
10-15 min.   Quick Candies, p.279; Carob Graham Crackers,
             p.280; Applesauce, p.290; Popcorn, p.292;
             Fresh fruit with carob sauce, p.296; Snacks to
             Go, p.279. With pre-preparation, Frozen Fruit
             Desserts, pp.293-295.

## RECIPES CHILDREN LOVE, & ALLERGY FREE RECIPES

### RECIPES CHILDREN LOVE

Oatmeal,133.
Pancakes,142-143.
Eggs,146-147.
Muffins,127-128.
Zucchini Bread,125.
Banana Bread,124.
Gingerbread,126.
Granola,138-140.
Apple Sauce,290.
Rehydrated Fruit,290.
Smoothies,158-159.
Fresh Vegetable Juices,
    pp.160-161.
Fresh Fruit
Nut/Seed milks,154-156.
"Soft Drinks",165
Sunburgers,230-231.
Sprouts,109-117.
All American Pizza,229.
Sandwiches
Vegetable Pies,229,235.

Lentil/Walnut Burgers,273.
Rice/Cheese/Nut Loaf,253.
Steamed Vegetables,224.
Vegetable Casserole,228.
Grain Salad,257-260.
Potato Pancakes,238.
Baked Squash,236.
Baked Potato,238.
Raw Vegetables
    Plus Dip,205-206.
Vegetable Soup,180.
Sweet Potato Soup,176,186.
Potato Leek Soup,188.
Curried Chicken,216.
Coq au Vin,215.
Fish Orientale,220.
Broiled Fish,220.
Spaghetti with sauce,210.
Tomatoes Provincale,237.
Anything from Snacks
    and Desserts,277-296.

### ALLERGY FREE TIPS AND RECIPES

(Most recipes in this book are dairy and wheat free.)

WHEAT FREE:
Conversion Tips for Using Other Grain Flours in Place of
    Wheat, 64-65.
Essene Bread,121.
2-Slice Bread,123.
Corn Muffins,127.
Gingerbread,126.
Almond Torte,285.

Rye Bread,122.
Millet Banana Bread,124.
Applesauce Muffins,128.
Carob Brownies,281.

EGG FREE:
Conversion Tips for Substituting eggs in a recipe with
    other ingredients,66.

DAIRY FREE:
In place of cow's milk, use:
Nut Milk,154-156.
Grain Water,152,166-167.
Soy Milk, store bought.

TOMATO FREE TOMATO SAUCE,211.

******** ALPHABETICAL INDEX ********